STUDY GUIDE
GERIATRIC PSYCHIATRY

A Companion to
The American Psychiatric Publishing
Textbook of Geriatric Psychiatry,
Fourth Edition

STUDY GUIDE TO
GERIATRIC PSYCHIATRY

A Companion to
The American Psychiatric Publishing
Textbook of Geriatric Psychiatry,
Fourth Edition

Robert E. Hales, M.D., M.B.A.

Joe P. Tupin Professor and Chair, Department of Psychiatry and Behavioral Sciences
University of California, Davis School of Medicine
Director, UC Davis Health System Behavioral Health Center
Director, UC Davis Sierra Health Foundation MD/MBA Fellowship Program
Medical Director, Mental Health Services, County of Sacramento
Sacramento, California

Narriman C. Shahrokh

Chief Administrative Officer, Department of Psychiatry and Behavioral Sciences
University of California, Davis School of Medicine
Sacramento, California

Dan G. Blazer, M.D., Ph.D.

J.P. Gibbons Professor of Psychiatry and Behavioral Sciences
and Professor of Community and Family Medicine
Duke University Medical Center
Durham, North Carolina

David C. Steffens, M.D., M.H.S.

Professor of Psychiatry and Head, Division of Geriatric Psychiatry
Duke University Medical Center
Durham, North Carolina

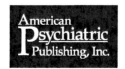

American Psychiatric Publishing, Inc.

Washington, DC
London, England

If you would like to buy between 25 and 99 copies of this or any other APPI title, you are eligible for a 20% discount; please contact APPI Customer Service at appi@psych.org or 800-368-5777. If you wish to buy 100 or more copies of the same title, please email us at bulksales@psych.org for a price quote.

Manufactured in the United States of America on acid-free paper
13 12 11 10 09   5 4 3 2 1

ISBN 978-1-58562-352-5
First Edition

Typeset in Revival BT and Adobe's The Mix

American Psychiatric Publishing, Inc.
1000 Wilson Boulevard
Arlington, VA 22209-3901
www.appi.org

Contents

Answer Guide

Preface

The purpose of this study guide is to provide individuals who have purchased the *American Psychiatric Publishing Textbook of Geriatric Psychiatry*, Fourth Edition, an opportunity to evaluate their understanding of the material contained in the textbook. Whenever possible, the selected questions coincide with the major clinical points summarized at the end of each chapter. However, every effort is made to select those questions of most relevance to psychiatrists who see patients in a variety of clinical practice settings.

We encourage the readers of the textbook to answer the questions after reading each chapter. The format for the questions is similar to what candidates would expect to encounter when taking the specialty-certifying examination in geriatric psychiatry. At the end of the study guide, the questions are repeated along with detailed answers. The answer section includes an explanation of the correct response for each question, as well as an explanation, in most cases, for why the other responses were incorrect.

An online version is available in addition to the printed study guide. Psychiatrists who wish to earn continuing medical education credits may purchase the online version and obtain CME credit by completing it.

We hope you will find the study guide a useful addition to the *Textbook of Geriatric Psychiatry*. Our goal is to have an assessment instrument that is helpful for your understanding of the material and for clarification of important concepts. Although the questions are reviewed numerous times, both by the authors and by editors at American Psychiatric Publishing, Inc., occasionally an incorrect response may be included. If this is the case, we would appreciate your notifying the publisher of the error so it can be corrected in the online version of the self-assessment examination. If you have other suggestions concerning this study guide, please e-mail Dr. Hales at rehales@ucdavis.edu.

Best of luck with your self-examination.

Robert E. Hales, M.D., M.B.A.
Narriman C. Shahrokh
Sacramento, CA

Chapter 1

The Myth, History, and Science of Aging

Select the single best response for each question.

1.1 A number of scientists have studied human tissues and cells to investigate the process of aging. Which of the following investigators became convinced that some human cells grown in culture were immortal?

    A. Hayflick and Moorhead.
    B. Medvedev.
    C. Carrel.
    D. Lepeshinskaya.
    E. Bacon.

1.2 A number of theories of aging have been proposed by various investigators. Which one of the following types of theories holds that aging is the result of sequential switching on and off of certain genes, and that defects develop during this switching on and off?

    A. Error theories.
    B. Somatic mutation theories.
    C. Cellular-based theories.
    D. Program theories.
    E. Exhaustion theories.

1.3 Processes of aging that are associated with random changes, such as cell loss or mutation, are part of which of the following theories?

    A. Stochastic theory.
    B. The master clock.
    C. Deliberate biological programming.
    D. The telomere theory.
    E. The free radical theory.

1.4 There are a number of genetic syndromes that are linked with premature aging. Although all of these are quite rare, one is characterized by dwarfism, physical immaturity, pseudosenility, and hypermetabolism. The affected individuals usually die in their mid-teens of coronary heart disease. Which of the following is this disorder?

    A. Werner's syndrome.
    B. Hutchinson-Gilford syndrome.
    C. Down syndrome.
    D. Laurence-Seip syndrome.
    E. Cockayne's syndrome.

1.5 There are a number of sex differences in longevity. Which of the following statements concerning men and women is *false*?

    A. Before 1900, in those nations where data are available, there were slightly more older men than older women.
    B. In 2007, the life expectancy for females was 7 years longer than for males in Japan.
    C. The single most important cause of higher mortality in males than females is an increased incidence of cigarette smoking in males.
    D. In non-industrial societies, women are more vulnerable to infectious diseases than men, leading to higher mortality rates.
    E. In the United States there are equal numbers of males and females born.

1.6 A number of social theories of aging have been proposed. Proponents of one theoretical approach maintain that older people tend to behave according to a pattern that has been established before late life. Which theory does this describe?

    A. The disengagement theory.
    B. The activity theory.
    C. The continuity theory.
    D. The age stratification theory.
    E. The life events and stress theory.

Chapter 2

Demography and Epidemiology of Psychiatric Disorders in Late Life

Select the single best response for each question.

2.1   Which of the following demographic statistics concerning older adults is *true*?

   A. In 2000, approximately 12.3 million persons in the United States were age 65 or older.
   B. In 2000, the number of "oldest old" or persons age 85 or older was 2.1 million.
   C. Nursing home residence has increased in recent years.
   D. The life expectancy in the United States for women increased from 48.3 years in 1900 to 80.4 years in 2004.
   E. The percentage of men 70 or older in the labor force increased from 20.8% in 1903 to 32.8% in 2003.

2.2   Diagnostic categories that approximate true disease processes should have several characteristics. Which of the following is *not* one of these characteristics?

   A. A category should predict the outcome of a disorder.
   B. A category should reflect underlying biological reality.
   C. The classification scheme should identify persons who would not be responsive to a specific therapeutic intervention.
   D. Laboratory studies should eventually validate a diagnostic category.
   E. A category should be distinguished on the basis of patterns of symptomatology.

2.3   One of the landmark studies of the prevalence of psychiatric disorders in the United States was the Epidemiologic Catchment Area (ECA) survey. Which of the following statements concerning the ECA is *true*?

   A. The ECA sought to determine the prevalence of specific psychiatric disorders in community, but not institutional settings.
   B. Data were collected in three communities.
   C. The most prevalent disorder in individuals 65 or older was depressive disorder.
   D. The diagnoses were based on DSM-IV criteria.
   E. A total of 12.3% of those 65 or older met criteria for one or more psychiatric disorders in the month prior to the interview.

2.4   The prevalence of psychiatric disorders in community populations of older adults (age 55 or older) is relatively consistent across most disorders. Which of the following prevalence rates is *false*?

   A. The prevalence rate of major depression generally ranged from 1%–3%.
   B. The prevalence of individual disorders was highest for panic disorder (3%–10%).
   C. The prevalence of any anxiety disorder in the ECA studies was 5.5%.
   D. The prevalence of anxiety disorders is higher than that of major depression.
   E. The prevalence of alcohol abuse/dependence was low (0.1%–1.5%).

2.5 Which of the following statements concerning psychiatric disorders in older adults is **true**?

    A. Psychiatric disorders are found at a higher prevalence among the elderly than at other stages of the life cycle.

    B. DSM-IV-TR provides age-specific categories for elderly persons, similar to children.

    C. The prevalence of major depression in nursing homes or long-term care facilities (1%–3%) is no different from prevalence in community samples of older adults.

    D. Suicide mortality is positively correlated with age.

    E. Older women are less likely to die from suicide than young women.

2.6 A number of genetic and environmental factors may increase the prevalence or age of onset of Alzheimer's disease in seniors. Which of the following statements concerning these factors is **false**?

    A. Persons who are first-degree relatives of someone with Alzheimer's disease are more likely to develop the disease earlier in life.

    B. A family history for dementia was positive for many more patients with Alzheimer's disease compared with individuals who were cognitively intact.

    C. Genetic research in Alzheimer's disease has focused on the *APOE*E2* allele.

    D. An association between early-onset Alzheimer's disease and Down syndrome has been reported.

    E. Retrospective studies of the association between head trauma and Alzheimer's disease have found a higher risk of Alzheimer's disease in persons with a history of head trauma.

Chapter 3

Physiological and Clinical Considerations of Geriatric Patient Care

Select the single best response for each question.

3.1 You have a 70-year-old physician patient whom you have treated for a number of years with psychodynamic psychotherapy. She notices that her vision is somewhat impaired around twilight. She asks you about any age-related changes to the eye that may have occurred. Your explanation of age-related changes to the eye that may be impairing her vision at twilight includes all of the following *except*

    A. The pupil becomes more miotic with age.
    B. There is increased curvature of the lens.
    C. The blood vessels of the iris have increased rigidity.
    D. The dilator muscle fibers atrophy.
    E. The lens thickens.

3.2 The heart and blood vessels in the aging patient undergo significant anatomic and physiologic alterations. Which of the following is an example of these changes that occur with aging?

    A. The blood vessels become more distensible.
    B. The intima undergoes significant hypoplasia.
    C. Systolic blood pressure is lower.
    D. There is a decrease in pulse wave velocity.
    E. The cushioning effect of the arterial system is adversely altered.

3.3 Your 72-year-old male patient asks you what he could do to improve his respiratory functioning because he has noticed a marked decrease in his respiratory capacity. Although you tell him that respiratory decline cannot be reversed, you recommend which of the following, which has been shown to slow the rate of decline?

    A. Moderate alcohol intake.
    B. Improved sleep hygiene.
    C. Exercise training.
    D. Dietary changes.
    E. Beta-adrenergic blocking agents.

3.4 Which of the following changes in endocrine function occurs in elderly patients?

    A. Basal antidiuretic hormone (ADH) levels are normal to increased.
    B. Basal corticotropin levels are decreased.
    C. Aldosterone levels are increased.
    D. Growth hormone levels continue to rise and peak at age 70.
    E. Thyroid function declines significantly leading to an increased risk of hypothyroidism.

3.5 Aging has no effect upon which of the following pharmacokinetic properties?

   A. Volume of distribution.
   B. Renal clearance rate.
   C. Hepatic drug clearance.
   D. Absorption.
   E. Elimination half-life.

3.6 Falls in the elderly are unfortunately quite common and are usually multifactorial in origin. By encouraging a patient to improve conditioning and strength through exercise, you are focusing on altering a(n)

   A. Extrinsic factor.
   B. Situational factor.
   C. Psychological factor.
   D. Environmental factor.
   E. Intrinsic factor.

3.7 A patient who complains of increased urinary frequency, nocturia, and varying amounts of leakage has which form of established urinary incontinence?

   A. Stress incontinence.
   B. Urge incontinence.
   C. Bladder outlet obstruction.
   D. Detrusor underactivity.
   E. Overflow incontinence.

3.8 In men with overflow incontinence, which of the following medications is sometimes prescribed?

   A. Oxybutynin.
   B. Propanolamine.
   C. Alpha-adrenergic blocking agents.
   D. Imipramine.
   E. Tolterodine.

Chapter 4

Neuroanatomy, Neurophysiology, and Neuropathology of Aging

Select the single best response for each question.

4.1 A 67-year-old patient reports a sudden onset of the inability to rotate or tilt his head. You refer him to a neurologist who reports a lesion affecting only the patient's cranial nerve. Which cranial nerve has been affected?

A. CN VII.
B. CN IX.
C. CN X.
D. CN XI.
E. CN XII.

4.2 Which of the following brain stem structures innervates virtually the entire forebrain and is composed of norepinephrine-rich neuronal bodies?

A. Substantia nigra.
B. Ventral tegmental area.
C. Locus coeruleus.
D. Dorsal raphe nucleus.
E. Periaqueductal gray.

4.3 Which of the following brain structures is located at the base of the cerebrum and coordinates endocrine, autonomic, and somatic motor responses to maintain physiological homeostasis?

A. Hypothalamus.
B. Thalamus.
C. Cerebellum.
D. Pons.
E. Medulla.

4.4 Deep in the cerebrum are several nuclei constituting the basal ganglia. A multitude of names are given to these structures in various combinations. Which of the following structures comprise the dorsal striatum?

A. Caudate and globus pallidus.
B. Putamen and globus pallidus.
C. Pallidum.
D. Ventral striatum.
E. Caudate and putamen.

4.5 Which of the following structures provides cholinergic innervation to virtually the entire neocortex?

    A. Ventral striatopallidum.
    B. Basal nucleus.
    C. Extended amygdala.
    D. Stria terminalis.
    E. Septal nuclei.

4.6 The cerebral cortex can be classified in several different ways. Which category of cortex is characterized by a poorly developed inner granular layer and prominent pyramidal cell layers?

    A. Allocortex.
    B. Association cortex.
    C. Agranular cortex.
    D. Neocortex.
    E. Koniocortex.

4.7 The limbic system is an open system of cortical and subcortical structures with extensive interconnections throughout the central nervous system. Which of the following is one of the cortical limbic structures?

    A. Mamillary nuclei.
    B. Hypothalamus.
    C. Amygdaloid complex.
    D. Hippocampus.
    E. Ventral striatum.

4.8 The EEG of a healthy awake adult is dominated by frequencies in which range?

    A. Delta.
    B. Theta.
    C. Alpha.
    D. Beta.
    E. Chi.

4.9 The brain is composed of neurons and supporting cells and structures. Which of the following supporting elements is a complex lipoprotein that serves to protect axonal processes and to facilitate neurotransmission?

    A. Myelin.
    B. Astrocytes.
    C. Oligodendroglia.
    D. Ependyma.
    E. Glia.

4.10 Many neurodegenerative processes cause abnormal aggregation of proteins leading to the formation of tangle inclusions in neuronal and glia cells. These proteins are almost entirely made of the protein tubulin and comprise which of the following specialized cell structures?

    A. Lysosomes.
    B. Microtubules.
    C. Lipfusion granules.
    D. Neurofilaments.
    E. Microfilaments.

C h a p t e r   5

Chemical Messengers

Select the single best response for each question.

5.1   Acetylcholine (ACh) acts through a family of muscarinic ACh receptors. Which muscarinic (M) receptor is the most abundant receptor in the neocortex and hippocampus tissue?

    A. M_1.
    B. M_2.
    C. M_3.
    D. M_4.
    E. M_5.

5.2   Which of the following is the major excitatory neurotransmitter in the human brain?

    A. Acetylcholine.
    B. Glutamate.
    C. Gamma-aminobutyric acid.
    D. Dopamine.
    E. Norepinephrine.

5.3   The family of serotonin receptors is separated into seven subgroups based on their sequence identities and related functions, with no fewer than 14 individual receptors. Which of the following receptors are decreased by 10% or more per decade in elderly people as compared to young subjects?

    A. 5-HT_{1F}.
    B. 5-HT_{1E}.
    C. 5-HT_{1D}.
    D. 5-HT_{1B}.
    E. 5-HT_{1A}.

5.4   Which of the following neurotransmitters is a substrate for both monoamine oxidase (MAO) and catechol O-methyltransferase (COMT) yielding the metabolic products homovanillic acid dihydroxyphenylacetic acid?

    A. Serotonin.
    B. Acetylcholine.
    C. Glutamate.
    D. Dopamine.
    E. Histamine.

5.5 Which of the following neurotransmitters produces release of stress hormones such as corticotropin-releasing factor and arginine vasopressin?

    A. Serotonin.
    B. Acetylcholine.
    C. Glutamate.
    D. Dopamine.
    E. Histamine.

Chapter 6

Genetics

Select the single best response for each question.

6.1 Among the fundamental insights to arise from the Human Genome Project is that

    A. The number of genes identified encompassed approximately 80% of all DNA.
    B. The number of genes was considerably more than expected, currently estimated as 400,000–500,000.
    C. The number and function of genes varies widely across mammalian species.
    D. The largest proportion of variation within humans and in comparison to other primates is due to structural variations, deletions, and duplications of segments of chromosomes.
    E. The silent or noncoding DNA is translated into complex proteins, similar to the genes.

6.2 Diseases caused by genomic rearrangements that result in an altered number of gene copies are often referred to as

    A. Single-nucleotide polymorphisms (SNPs).
    B. Genomic disorders.
    C. Noncoding (nc) DNA errors.
    D. Noncoding (nc) RNA errors.
    E. Gene transcription disorders.

6.3 An example of a phenotype that arises from a single-gene disorder is

    A. Early-onset Alzheimer's disease.
    B. Late-onset Alzheimer's disease.
    C. Major depressive disorders.
    D. Bipolar disorders.
    E. Schizophrenia.

6.4 A patient of yours is concerned about her risk of developing late-onset Alzheimer's disease, since her 85-year-old mother has this disorder. What do you tell her is her actual predicted risk of developing Alzheimer's disease?

    A. 31%–40%.
    B. 26%–30%.
    C. 20%–25%.
    D. 15%–19%.
    E. 9%–14%.

6.5 The one gene with a clearly established relationship to late-onset Alzheimer's disease is

    A. Amyloid precursor protein gene (*APP*).
    B. Presenilin-1 (*PS1*).
    C. Apolipoprotein E, ε4 allele (*APOE*E4*).
    D. Presenilin-2 (*PS2*).
    E. Apolipoprotein E, ε2 allele (*APOE*E2*).

Chapter 7

Psychological Aspects of Normal Aging

Select the single best response for each question.

7.1 Which of the following primary mental abilities declines last with aging but also shows a steeper decline than other abilities from the 70s to the 80s?

    A. Numeric ability.
    B. Inductive reasoning.
    C. Verbal meaning.
    D. Spatial orientation.
    E. Word fluency.

7.2 At what age will the average older adult's primary mental abilities fall below the middle range of performance for young adults?

    A. 40s.
    B. 50s.
    C. 60s.
    D. 70s.
    E. 80s.

7.3 Three studies have examined the predictors of the number of days of survival beyond 100 years. Which of the following was a common variable in all three studies that predicted longer survival?

    A. Gender.
    B. Father's age of death.
    C. Residential condition.
    D. Cognitive status.
    E. Nutritional sufficiency.

7.4 For the clinical psychiatrist, the contributions of neuroimaging research to cognitive changes associated with aging lead to all of the following conclusions *except*

    A. Cognitive change occurs throughout late adulthood.
    B. Some decline in perceptual speed and fluid abilities will be evident only in individuals with early signs of dementias.
    C. Significant changes in brain structure and function may occur in individuals without noticeable cognitive impairment.
    D. Age-related cognitive decline may be minimized to the degree that cardiovascular disease and other comorbidities can be avoided.
    E. The brain is constantly adapting and this adaptation is expressed in measures of older adults' brain function and behavioral measures of cognitive performance.

7.5 Recent research suggests that personality may in fact change over time. Which of the following changes has been reported to occur with aging?

    A. Decrease in neuroticism.
    B. Increase in extraversion.
    C. Decrease in agreeableness.
    D. Increase in openness.
    E. Decrease in conscientiousness.

7.6 A patient asks you whether there are certain personality traits that may predict shorter life spans or premature mortality. Which of the following is such a personality characteristic?

    A. Agreeableness.
    B. Conscientiousness.
    C. Pessimism.
    D. Openness to experiences.
    E. Optimism.

Chapter 8

Social and Economic Factors Related to Psychiatric Disorders in Late Life

Select the single best response for each question.

8.1 A consensual model of the precursors of psychiatric disorders has emerged from the social science and social psychiatry literature. The model is composed of a series of stages. Each of the following is one of these stages *except*

   A. Social integration.
   B. Early events and achievements.
   C. Biological variables.
   D. Provoking agents and copying efforts.
   E. Later events and achievements.

8.2 A number of demographic variables have been examined to determine their association with psychiatric disorder in the elderly. Age and gender are two factors that are related to the risk of psychiatric disorders. Which of the following statements concerning age is *true?*

   A. In studies of age differences within the older population, depressive symptoms are lowest among the oldest.
   B. Older adults report levels of depressive symptoms lower than those reported by younger and middle-aged adults.
   C. Some studies have found lower rates of psychiatric symptoms among older adults in comparison to younger adults.
   D. There is a lower lifetime prevalence of depression among older adults.
   E. Older women report lower levels of psychiatric symptoms than men.

8.3 Occupation, income, and marriage are important life conditions related to the development of psychiatric disorders. Which of the following statements concerning these life conditions is *false?*

   A. Low income is a risk factor for depressive symptoms.
   B. Retirement increases the risk of developing a psychiatric disorder.
   C. Marital status is weakly associated with psychiatric morbidity.
   D. Remarried women are at significantly higher risk of depression than women married only once.
   E. The unmarried typically report significantly more symptoms of depression than the married.

8.4 A primary protective factor for the development of psychiatric disorders has been social support. There are several dimensions of social support. One dimension is defined as the specific tangible services provided by families and friends. Which of the following is the dimension?

   A. Social network.
   B. Perceptions of social support.
   C. Informational support.
   D. Level of interaction with family and friends.
   E. Instrumental support.

8.5 Compared with current cohorts of older adults, younger adults now are

    A. Less likely to marry.
    B. Less likely to marry for the first time at later ages.
    C. Less likely to divorce.
    D. More likely to have children.
    E. Less likely to have fewer children.

8.6 In reviewing a number of studies to determine the likelihood of an older adult recovering from depression, you come to several conclusions about factors that may contribute to a poorer outcome. Which of the following factors is associated with a higher likelihood of an older adult's recovering from depression?

    A. Being older.
    B. Being treated in the general medical sector.
    C. Being male.
    D. The recent occurrence of significant life events.
    E. None of the above.

8.7 There are a number of reasons why the majority of psychiatric disorders among older adults are treated in the general medical sector. Which of the following is *not* one of these reasons?

    A. Older persons prefer to receive treatment from their primary care physicians.
    B. Medication is greatly preferred over psychotherapy.
    C. Primary care physicians do not refer older patients with psychiatric disorders to mental health professionals.
    D. Older adults are concerned about the stigma of having a psychiatric disorder and needing care.
    E. Older adults have more negative attitudes towards mental health professionals.

Chapter 9

The Psychiatric Interview of Older Adults

Select the single best response for each question.

9.1 In gathering information from elderly patients concerning their present illness, you should assess their function and change in function. Two important parameters for this type of assessment are not normally included in the assessment of physical and psychiatric illness in younger adults. One of these parameters is social functioning. What is the other?

    A. Alcohol use.
    B. Current medications.
    C. Employment.
    D. Activities of daily living.
    E. Educational achievement.

9.2 A primary goal of the clinician as an advocate for the psychiatrically ill older adult is to facilitate family support. Areas that are important to evaluate include all of the following *except*

    A. Whether a family member has a similar psychiatric disorder.
    B. Tolerance by the family of specific behavior related to the psychiatric disorder.
    C. The tangible services that may be provided by the family.
    D. Availability of family members.
    E. Perceptions of family support by the older patient.

9.3 Testing the memory of an older patient is an important component of the mental status examination. Asking the older person to repeat a word, phrase, or series of numbers assesses which component of memory?

    A. Registration.
    B. Retention.
    C. Immediate recall.
    D. Orientation.
    E. Distant memory.

9.4 A number of rating scales have been used to screen for depression in seniors. Which of the following is an interviewer-rated scale that does *not* include many of the somatic symptoms that tend to be more common in older adults?

    A. Center for Epidemiologic Studies Depression Scale (CES-D).
    B. Montgomery-Åsberg Rating Scale for Depression.
    C. Beck Depression Inventory (BDI).
    D. Geriatric Depression Scale (GDS).
    E. Hamilton Rating Scale for Depression (Ham-D).

9.5 Which of the following general assessment scales produces functional impairment ratings in five areas: mental health, physical health, social functioning, economic functioning, and activities of daily living?

    A. Global Assessment of Functioning Scale.
    B. Geriatric Mental State Schedule.
    C. Psychiatric Status Schedule.
    D. Comprehensive Assessment and Referral Evaluation.
    E. Older Americans Resources and Services (OARS) Multidimensional Functional Assessment Questionnaire.

9.6 In interviewing an older patient, psychiatrists may apply a variety of techniques to improve communication. In general, which of the following techniques should *not* be used in older adults?

    A. Speak clearly and slowly, since many seniors have hearing difficulties.
    B. Take a position near the older person.
    C. Address the person by surname to demonstrate respect.
    D. Avoid silent pauses, since elders get uncomfortable with silence.
    E. Allow the senior enough time to respond to questions.

Chapter 10

Use of the Laboratory in the Diagnostic Workup of Older Adults

Select the single best response for each question.

10.1 You are treating an 83-year-old patient for depression and she develops fatigue, nausea, dizziness, gait disturbances, forgetfulness, confusion, lethargy, and muscle cramps. You obtain a general chemistry panel, and her serum sodium concentration is 120 mEq/L. What psychotropic medication has been reported to produce this condition in the elderly?

    A. Bupropion.
    B. Selective serotonin reuptake inhibitors.
    C. Depakote.
    D. Venlafaxine.
    E. Tricyclic antidepressants.

10.2 You are asked to evaluate a 79-year-old man who was hospitalized on the general medical service for evaluation of mental status changes associated with malnutrition. You recommend to the medical team that they order a serum homocysteine level. The resident asks why the order is necessary. All of the following answers are true *except*

    A. Hyperhomocysteinemia is prevalent in the elderly.
    B. High levels of homocysteine can be attributed to an inadequate supply of B_{12} and folate.
    C. Hyperhomocysteinemia is associated with cognitive dysfunction.
    D. High levels of homocysteine have been associated with an increased risk for occlusive vascular disease, thrombosis, and stroke.
    E. Vitamin supplementation to reduce plasma homocysteine has been shown in numerous studies to improve cognition.

10.3 In a community psychiatry clinic, you see for the first time a 78-year-old patient who has been treated for a number of years with thioridazine. You immediately decide to order an electrocardiogram (ECG). What ECG changes are you particularly concerned about?

    A. Atrioventricular block.
    B. Sinoatrial block.
    C. QTc prolongation.
    D. PR internal prolongation.
    E. Prolonged QRS complex.

10.4 When used to examine brain structures, computed tomography (CT) is an effective radiographic technique. However, it does have limitations. Which of the following is a major limitation?

    A. It cannot demonstrate bone abnormalities such as skull fractures.
    B. It is not effective in detecting subdural hematomas.
    C. It is ineffective in showing the mass effect from various lesions.
    D. It does not visualize posterior fossa structures well because of surrounding bone.
    E. It cannot demonstrate ventricular enlargement.

10.5 When compared with CT imaging, magnetic resonance imaging (MRI) has advantages and disadvantages. All of the following are disadvantages of MRI, as compared to CT, *except*

    A. Radiation is used.
    B. The procedure takes longer.
    C. It is usually more costly.
    D. The device must be housed in an area devoid of iron.
    E. Patients cannot carry or wear certain metals or have them embedded in their bodies.

Chapter 11

Neuropsychological Assessment of Dementia

Select the single best response for each question.

11.1 Age-related cognitive changes are manifested in the decline in a number of tasks or abilities. Which of the following cognitive processes are less susceptible to age?

    A. Motor responses.
    B. Crystallized skills.
    C. Reaction times.
    D. Fluid abilities.
    E. Retrieval functions.

11.2 In the early stages of Alzheimer's disease, the medial temporal lobe is most affected, leading to impairment of which of the following cognitive processes?

    A. Recent memory.
    B. Expressive language.
    C. Visuospatial function.
    D. Higher executive control.
    E. Semantic knowledge.

11.3 Which of the following dementias is characterized by early fluctuations in cognition and attention, recurrent and persistent visual hallucinations, and extrapyramidal motor symptoms?

    A. Alzheimer's disease.
    B. Frontotemporal lobar dementia (FTLD).
    C. Dementia with Lewy bodies (DLB).
    D. Parkinson's disease dementia (PDD).
    E. Vascular dementia.

11.4 Which of the following dementias is characterized by prominent early changes in behavior, personality, or language, as opposed to impairments in memory and other aspects of cognition?

    A. Alzheimer's disease.
    B. Frontotemporal lobar dementia.
    C. Lewy body dementia.
    D. Parkinson's disease dementia.
    E. Vascular dementia.

11.5 PDD and DLB may be distinguished from Alzheimer's disease by which of the following symptoms that normally occur early on in both PDD and DLB?

    A. Selective recent memory disturbance.
    B. Expressive language defects.
    C. Semantic knowledge impairments.
    D. Impaired judgment.
    E. Visual spatial disturbances.

Chapter 12

Delirium

Select the single best response for each question.

12.1 Key clinical features of delirium that are assessed by the Confusion Assessment Method (CAM) include all of the following *except*

    A. Inattention.
    B. Stable course.
    C. Acute onset.
    D. Disorganized thinking.
    E. Altered level of consciousness.

12.2 Several neurotransmitters have been implicated in the mechanism of delirium. The most frequently considered neurotransmitter, for which there is the most evidence, is

    A. Acetylcholine.
    B. Norepinephrine.
    C. Glutamate.
    D. Melatonin.
    E. Dopamine.

12.3 Which of the following is the leading risk factor for development of delirium?

    A. Advanced age.
    B. Male gender.
    C. Vision or hearing impairments.
    D. Alcohol abuse or dependence.
    E. Dementia.

12.4 A predictive risk model that identifies predisposing factors for delirium has been developed for hospitalized older patients at discharge. Which of the following is *not* one of these risk factors?

    A. Use of physical restraints during delirium.
    B. Functional impairment.
    C. High comorbidity.
    D. Auditory impairment.
    E. Dementia.

12.5 The key diagnostic feature(s) present in delirium but not dementia is/are

    A. Visual hallucinations.
    B. Cognitive impairment.
    C. Acute onset.
    D. Memory disturbance.
    E. Delusions.

12.6 First-line nonpharmacological treatment approaches to delirium should **not** include

    A. Frequent eye contact.
    B. Clear instructions.
    C. Assessment and correction of sensory deficits.
    D. Verbal reorienting strategies.
    E. Use of physical restraints.

Chapter 13

Dementia and Milder Cognitive Syndromes

Select the single best response for each question.

13.1 You have a 65-year-old patient who presents with a clinical syndrome consisting of a measurable decline in memory with little effect on day-to-day functioning. Which of the following best describes this syndrome?

    A. Delirium.
    B. Dementia.
    C. Alzheimer's disease.
    D. Cognitive impairment not dementia (CIND).
    E. Mild cognitive impairment (MCI).

13.2 For the dementia syndrome to be present, key elements must be exhibited by the patient. Which of the following is *not* one of these key elements?

    A. Basic daily living activities must be impaired.
    B. The cognitive symptoms must represent a cognitive decline.
    C. The cognitive syndrome must be present in the absence of delirium.
    D. The person's daily functioning must be impaired.
    E. Only one area of cognition may be affected.

13.3 Traditionally, dementia is differentiated into cortical and subcortical subsyndromes. Which of the following areas of impairment is indicative of subcortical dementia?

    A. Amnesia.
    B. Apraxia.
    C. Dysexecutive.
    D. Aphasia.
    E. Agnosia.

13.4 Which of the following neuropsychiatric symptom clusters is indicative of loss of executive control?

    A. Spontaneous violence, intrusions, wandering.
    B. Sleep, sexual, or feeding disturbances.
    C. Delusions and hallucinations.
    D. Apathy, depression, anxiety, and irritability.
    E. None of the above.

13.5 The Mini-Mental State Examination (MMSE) is widely used as a screening instrument for dementia. What is its major limitation?

    A. It must be administered by individuals skilled in its use.
    B. It is unable to detect severe forms of dementia.
    C. It is time-consuming to administer.
    D. It has limitations in evaluating executive control function.
    E. It does not provide a numerical score.

13.6 Which of the following dementia syndromes is the second most common form of dementia in persons under age 65, with a rate of occurrence that is close to that of Alzheimer's disease?

    A. Parkinson's disease dementia (PDD).
    B. Frontotemporal degeneration (FTD).
    C. Dementia with Lewy bodies (DLB).
    D. Dementia due to normal pressure hydrocephalus.
    E. Dementia due to prion diseases.

13.7 Which of the following cholinesterase inhibitors is available in patch form and has been approved by the U.S. Food and Drug Administration (FDA) to treat PDD?

    A. Huperzine.
    B. Tacrine.
    C. Donepezil.
    D. Galantamine.
    E. Rivastigmine.

Chapter 14

Movement Disorders

Select the single best response for each question.

14.1 Parkinsonism has been associated with the use of antipsychotic medications. Which of the following agents is *least* likely to produce parkinsonism symptoms?

    A. Haloperidol.
    B. Olanzapine.
    C. Quetiapine.
    D. Risperidone.
    E. Thioridazine.

14.2 Parkinson's disease is a chronic, progressive, neurodegenerative illness that produces a constellation of motoric symptoms. Which of the following symptoms usually does *not* occur in Parkinson's disease?

    A. Rigidity.
    B. Bradykinesia.
    C. Postural instability.
    D. Intention tremor.
    E. Hypomimia.

14.3 There are a number of motor complications of Parkinson's disease. Which of the following symptoms is usually secondary to medications used to treat Parkinson's disease?

    A. Retropulsion.
    B. On-off phenomena.
    C. Postural instability.
    D. Freezing of gait.
    E. Festination.

14.4 You have a 72-year-old male patient who currently is on no medications and was recently diagnosed with Parkinson's disease by a neurologist. The most effective pharmacologic treatment is the administration of which of the following classes of medications?

    A. Anticholinergic agent.
    B. Monoamine oxidase B inhibitor.
    C. Dopamine agonist.
    D. Catechol O-methyltransferase (COMT) inhibitor.
    E. Dopamine precursor.

14.5 Which of the following movement disorders produces myoclonic, apraxic, rigid, akinetic movements and alien hand syndrome, in which one hand seems to have a mind of its own?

A. Cortical-basal ganglionic degeneration (CBGD).
B. Frontotemporal dementia.
C. Multiple system atrophy.
D. Progressive supranuclear palsy.
E. Normal pressure hydrocephalus.

14.6 There are a number of hyperkinetic movement disorders. Which of the following consists of rhythmic oscillations across a joint resulting from involuntary, alternating activation of agonist and antagonist muscles?

A. Chorea.
B. Dystonia.
C. Essential tremor.
D. Myoclonus.
E. Tics.

Chapter 15

Mood Disorders

Select the single best response for each question.

15.1 You diagnose major depression in a physically healthy 76-year-old woman and recommend to her antidepressant medication. She responds by saying, "What's the use? I've heard that antidepressants are not very effective in older people." You state that if seniors are treated with an adequate dose of an antidepressant for a sufficient period of time (at least 6–9 months) they may expect a recovery rate of approximately

A. 30%.
B. 40%.
C. 50%.
D. 60%.
E. 70%.

15.2 Factors associated with improved outcome in late-life depression include which of the following?

A. Family history of depression.
B. Male gender.
C. Introverted personality.
D. Substance abuse history.
E. Recent major life events.

15.3 Certain psychological factors may contribute to the onset of late-life depressive symptoms. All of the following factors have been reported by investigators to increase the likelihood or frequency of late-life depressive symptoms *except*

A. Hopelessness.
B. Cognitive distortions.
C. Acceptance.
D. Higher levels of mastery.
E. Rumination.

15.4 Adults are thought to acquire increased wisdom as they age. One group of investigators has operationalized wisdom and studied it in community samples. Which of the following criteria is *not* associated with increase wisdom?

A. Rich factual knowledge.
B. Absolute values and life priorities.
C. Life span contextualization.
D. Recognition and management of uncertainty.
E. Rich procedural knowledge.

15.5 An investigator compared the clinical, demographic, and social characteristics of psychotic and nonpsychotic depression in a large sample of elderly and younger hospitalized patients and found which of the following variables to be more common in psychotic depression?

    A. Good social support.
    B. Lack of suicidal ideation.
    C. Younger age.
    D. Cerebrovascular risk factors.
    E. Psychomotor agitation.

15.6 Minor, subsyndromal or subthreshold depression is commonly found in the elderly. Associations with subsyndromal depression are similar to those found in major depression, including all of the following *except*

    A. Unmarried status.
    B. Male gender.
    C. Poorer self-rated health.
    D. Perceived low social support.
    E. More disability days.

Chapter 16

Bipolar Disorder in Late Life

Select the single best response for each question.

16.1 The exact prevalence of bipolar disorder in late life is uncertain, but several large studies have reported prevalence rates in community samples to be

A. <0.5%
B. 1%–2%.
C. 3%–5%.
D. 6%–8%.
E. 9%–10%.

16.2 Which of the following variables is decreased or lower in older patients with bipolar disorder as compared with younger patients with bipolar disorder?

A. Depression as the initial episode of illness.
B. Medical comorbidity.
C. Substance abuse.
D. Mortality rates.
E. Dementia.

16.3 Evaluation of patients with late-life bipolar disorder reveals various patterns of presentation. Which of the following patterns is the most frequent in elderly patients with bipolar disorder?

A. Those who have never been recognized as having bipolar symptoms or who have been misdiagnosed.
B. Those who previously experienced only episodes of depression but have now switched to a manic episode.
C. Those who have never had bipolar disorder but develop mania due to a specific medical or neurological event.
D. Those who developed bipolar disorder earlier in life and are now seeking treatment.
E. Those who have never had bipolar disorder but develop mania for unknown reasons.

16.4 Hyperintense signals viewed on T2-weighted magnetic resonance imaging (MRI) images are among the earliest and most consistent neuroimaging findings in bipolar disorder. The presence of hyperintensities may be especially important in late-life bipolar disorder. MRI hyperintensities are associated with which of the following?

A. Longer hospital stays and more frequent rehospitalizations.
B. Risk modifiers for cognitive dysfunction in bipolar disorder.
C. Less reduction in manic symptoms during treatment.
D. An increasing role for these hyperintensities in bipolar cognitive impairment with increasing age.
E. All of the above.

16.5 Which of the following atypical antipsychotic agents is approved by the U.S. Food and Drug Administration (FDA) for the treatment of acute depression?

    A. Aripiprazole.
    B. Olanzapine.
    C. Ziprasidone.
    D. Risperidone.
    E. Quetiapine.

Chapter 17

Schizophrenia and Paranoid Disorders

Select the single best response for each question.

17.1 Recent data suggest that patients with late-onset schizophrenia, in comparison with early-onset patients, have a lower prevalence of

    A. The paranoid subtype.
    B. Persecutory delusions.
    C. Organized delusions.
    D. Auditory hallucinations.
    E. Negative symptoms.

17.2 Factors distinguishing patients with very-late-onset schizophrenia-like psychosis (VLOSLP), wherein the onset of psychosis is after age 60 years, from "true" schizophrenia patients, include all of the following *except*

    A. Lower genetic load.
    B. Less evidence of early childhood maladjustment.
    C. Less risk of tardive dyskinesia.
    D. A relative lack of thought disorder.
    E. More evidence of a neurodegenerative process.

17.3 Which of the following is the most common symptom in psychosis of Alzheimer's disease?

    A. Visual hallucinations.
    B. Delusions.
    C. Depression.
    D. Disorganization of speech and behavior.
    E. Auditory hallucinations.

17.4 In a consensus survey of 48 American experts on the treatment of older adults with late-life schizophrenia, the first-line medication treatment recommendation was

    A. Aripiprazole.
    B. Clozapine.
    C. Olanzapine.
    D. Quetiapine.
    E. Risperidone.

17.5 Recently the U.S. Food and Drug Administration (FDA) issued a black-box warning for the use of atypical antipsychotics in elderly dementia patients. Which adverse event was noted to occur at a higher rate in this patient population?

    A. Hyperlipidemia.
    B. Diabetes.
    C. Hypertension.
    D. Stroke.
    E. Weight gain.

17.6 In the National Institute of Mental Health Clinical Antipsychotic Trials of Intervention Effectiveness Alzheimer's disease (CATIE-AD) trial, which was the largest non-industry-sponsored trial of atypical antipsychotics for psychosis or agitation/aggression in people with dementia, which of the following agents was found to be better than placebo for the primary outcome measure?

    A. Aripiprazole.
    B. Olanzapine.
    C. Quetiapine.
    D. Risperidone.
    E. No agent.

Chapter 18

Anxiety Disorders

Select the single best response for each question.

18.1 All of the anxiety disorders are associated with some degree of avoidance and arousal. Based on these shared and distinct features, the anxiety disorders can be grouped into categories based on the nature of their phenomenology. Which of the following disorders is grouped into the fear category?

    A. Panic disorder.
    B. Acute stress disorder.
    C. Obsessive-compulsive disorder (OCD).
    D. Generalized anxiety disorder (GAD).
    E. Posttraumatic stress disorder (PTSD).

18.2 Several large epidemiological studies were published that included a large sample of elderly persons. Which of the following anxiety disorders is at least as common in late life as in younger adults?

    A. Obsessive-compulsive disorder.
    B. Generalized anxiety disorder.
    C. Panic disorder.
    D. Phobias (specific and social).
    E. Posttraumatic stress disorder.

18.3 The central feature of generalized anxiety disorder is

    A. Irritability.
    B. Fear.
    C. Worry.
    D. Arousal.
    E. Avoidance.

18.4 Which of the following has been reported to be the most common anxiety disorder in older African American patients?

    A. Generalized anxiety disorder.
    B. Panic disorder.
    C. Obsessive-compulsive disorder.
    D. Social phobia.
    E. Posttraumatic stress disorder.

18.5 Which of the following cognitive functions is usually not impaired in older patients with generalized anxiety disorder and may be even improved?

   A. Short-term memory.
   B. Recall.
   C. Long-term memory.
   D. Executive functioning.
   E. Delayed memory.

18.6 Depressed elderly patients with comorbid anxiety, in contrast to depressed elderly individuals without anxiety, usually have

   A. Lower risk of suicide.
   B. Reduced response rate to treatment.
   C. Shorter time to achieve a response to treatment.
   D. Fewer somatic symptoms.
   E. Less suicidal ideation.

Chapter 19

Somatoform Disorders

Select the single best response for each question.

19.1 The diagnostic feature of somatization disorder that is most difficult to establish in elderly patients is

  A. Pain at four or more sites.
  B. Physical complaints not fully explained by the medical workup.
  C. Onset prior to age 30.
  D. Relevant physical findings.
  E. Comorbid illness.

19.2 Undifferentiated somatoform disorder is defined by all of the following *except*

  A. Presence of one or more physical complaints.
  B. Symptoms last at least 6 months.
  C. Symptoms cannot be fully explained by appropriate medical workup.
  D. Symptoms result in considerable impairment.
  E. Symptoms include pain at four or more sites.

19.3 Which of the following is *not* a risk factor for conversion disorder?

  A. Being male.
  B. Physical abuse.
  C. Personality disorder.
  D. Other neurological illnesses.
  E. Sexual abuse.

19.4 What is the most common medical complaint in elderly persons?

  A. Dizziness.
  B. Pain.
  C. Constipation.
  D. Insomnia.
  E. Gait instability.

19.5 A number of factors have been associated with an increased risk for somatoform disorders. Which of the following is one of these factors?

  A. Male gender.
  B. Serious illness late in life.
  C. Higher educational level.
  D. Childhood abuse.
  E. High socioeconomic status.

Chapter 20

Sexual Disorders

Select the single best response for each question.

20.1 Which of the following is the first stage of the normal sexual response cycle?

    A. Plateau.
    B. Arousal.
    C. Orgasm.
    D. Desire.
    E. Resolution.

20.2 In women, the most significant changes in the sexual response cycle occur during menopause. Which of the following changes is caused by a decrease in testosterone?

    A. Atrophy of urogenital tissue.
    B. Less intense orgasms.
    C. Decreased libido.
    D. Decrease in vaginal size.
    E. Reduced vaginal lubrication.

20.3 As men age, which of the following sexual parameters increases instead of decreases?

    A. Volume of ejaculate.
    B. Refractory period.
    C. Libido.
    D. Bone and muscle mass.
    E. Frequency of erections.

20.4 In older men, especially those over the age of 70, the most common sexual disorder is

    A. Hypoactive sexual desire.
    B. Inhibited orgasm.
    C. Premature ejaculation.
    D. Sexual aversion.
    E. Erectile dysfunction.

20.5 You diagnose major depression in a 70-year-old man. He wants you to prescribe an antidepressant with the fewest sexual side effects. He is on no other medications and has no significant medical illnesses. Which of the following antidepressants do you recommend because it has the lowest rate of reported sexual dysfunction?

    A. Bupropion.
    B. Venlafaxine.
    C. Imipramine.
    D. Sertraline.
    E. Mirtazapine.

20.6 You prescribe an antidepressant for a 70-year-old man with major depression and no comorbid medical conditions. He calls you 2 weeks after starting the medication and states that his mood has improved greatly; however, he is experiencing some sexual side effects. What would be the most logical first step in addressing his sexual complaints?

    A. Encourage him to stop the medication over the weekend and encourage him to attempt sexual intercourse.
    B. Stop the medication and replace it with another antidepressant.
    C. Reduce the dose of the medication.
    D. Continue the medication and wait to see if the side effects decrease.
    E. Prescribe an antidote, such as sildenafil.

20.7 Hypoactive sexual desire in older women is caused by a number of psychological and physical factors. Which of the following is **not** one of these factors?

    A. Poor self-image.
    B. Increased estrogen production.
    C. Decreased free testosterone.
    D. Negative societal attitudes of sexuality in late life.
    E. Internalized negative images of sexuality in older persons.

Bereavement

Select the single best response for each question.

21.1 Numerous theoretical perspectives on the function and process of bereavement have been developed over the years. Who believed that any involuntary separation, including bereavement, gives rise to many forms of attachment behavior that reflect the person's desire to reunite with the lost person?

    A. Bierhals.
    B. Bowlby.
    C. Freud.
    D. Lindemann.
    E. Rosenblatt.

21.2 Several psychiatrists have proposed models of bereavement that involve phases or stages of reaction to the death of a loved one. Usually three stages are described. Which of the following is characteristic of the second or middle stage?

    A. Emotional numbness.
    B. Identity reconstruction.
    C. Cognitive confusion.
    D. Yearning and protest.
    E. Shock and disbelief.

21.3 Bonnano et al. collected data on 205 older adults several years prior to the death of their spouse and again at 6 and 18 months postloss. Five patterns of adjustment were identified based on pre- and postloss levels of adjustment. All of the following are among these patterns *except*

    A. Chronic grief.
    B. Resilience.
    C. Normal grief.
    D. Chronic depression.
    E. Denial.

21.4 A number of studies have been undertaken to identify elders at risk for negative outcomes after spousal loss. Which of the following variables is generally *not* associated with prolonged or complicated bereavement?

    A. Death by suicide.
    B. Intense negative emotions at 2 months postloss.
    C. Making sense of the loss.
    D. Unexpected death.
    E. Being a widower.

21.5 Of the following preloss variables in spouses, which one has **not** consistently been found to be a risk factor for complicated bereavement?

    A. More negative ratings of preloss relationship satisfaction.
    B. Preloss depression.
    C. Poor self-esteem.
    D. Inadequate coping skills.
    E. Lack of social support.

21.6 A number of psychological treatments for complicated bereavement have been studied. One such treatment is a 12-session phase-oriented strategy designed to help individuals work through emotional reactions to traumatic events. Which of the following is this treatment?

    A. Guided mourning.
    B. Cognitive-behavioral therapy.
    C. Time-limited psychodynamic psychotherapy.
    D. Interpersonal psychotherapy.
    E. Imaginal exposure.

Chapter 22

Sleep and Circadian Rhythm Disorders

Select the single best response for each question.

22.1 Extensive research has shown that marked changes in sleep and circadian rhythms accompany aging. Which of the following is an example of the changes that will occur with aging?

    A. Nocturnal sleep time increases.
    B. Time in stages 3 and 4 sleep increases.
    C. Nocturnal wake time increases.
    D. The amplitude of the sleep-wake cycle increases.
    E. Older adults tend to awaken at a later phase.

22.2 Which of the following primary sleep disorders is rare in adults age 60 years or older?

    A. Restless legs syndrome (RLS).
    B. Obstructive sleep apnea.
    C. Insomnia from depression.
    D. Periodic limb movement disorder (PLMD).
    E. Central sleep apnea.

22.3 Individuals with Alzheimer's disease experience a number of sleep changes. Which of the following is among the leading reasons that individuals with dementia become institutionalized?

    A. Increased arousals.
    B. Sundowning.
    C. More daytime naps.
    D. Decreased REM sleep.
    E. Decreased slow wave sleep.

22.4 The most troublesome symptom of sleep disturbance for patients with Parkinson's disease is

    A. Difficulty initiating sleep.
    B. Restless legs syndrome.
    C. Daytime fatigue.
    D. Difficulty maintaining sleep.
    E. Inability to turn over in bed.

22.5 Individuals with chronic obstructive pulmonary disease (COPD) have been found to have evidence of disturbed sleep. Which of the following statements concerning COPD and sleep is true?

    A. Daytime sleepiness does not routinely occur in COPD.
    B. Polysomnography is routinely indicated for COPD patients.
    C. The degree of sleep disturbance in COPD patients is related to the degree of hypoxemia.
    D. COPD patients who become hypoxemic at night are less likely to be hypoxemic during the day.
    E. Sleep apnea is more common in COPD patients than in the general population.

22.6 The most common reason given by elderly persons for difficulty in maintaining sleep is

    A. Restless legs syndrome.
    B. Depression.
    C. Periodic limb movement.
    D. Nocturia.
    E. Daytime naps.

22.7 You evaluate an elderly patient for depression and decide to begin her on an antidepressant because a significant problem for her has been sleep difficulties. She reports that she is able to fall asleep quickly, but that she awakens throughout the night. Which of the following agents would improve her ability to stay asleep?

    A. Ramelteon.
    B. Zaleplon.
    C. Eszopiclone.
    D. Zolpidem.
    E. Amitriptyline.

Chapter 23

Alcohol and Drug Problems

Select the single best response for each question.

23.1 When consumption of alcohol is at a level whereby adverse medical, psychological, or social consequences have occurred, older adults would be characterized as

    A. Alcohol dependent.
    B. Low-risk drinkers.
    C. Problem users.
    D. At-risk drinkers.
    E. Abstainers.

23.2 All of the following are beneficial effects of moderate alcohol consumption *except*

    A. Reduced risk of cardiovascular disease.
    B. Reduced risk of diabetes.
    C. Improved self-esteem.
    D. Lower odds of reporting physical limitations.
    E. Lower high-density lipoprotein serum level.

23.3 For a number of reasons, providers may fail to identify alcohol and substance use disorders in older patients. Which of the following is *not* one of the reasons for failure to identify these disorders?

    A. Mistaken belief that there are too many effective treatments.
    B. Misconception that older substance users must have a lifelong history of problem use.
    C. Difficulty in applying diagnostic criteria for substance use disorders to seniors.
    D. Lack of appreciation of the benefits of reduced substance use.
    E. Insufficient knowledge of the potential health impact of problem drinking.

23.4 The "gold standard" for assessing the quantity and frequency of alcohol and drug use is

    A. The timeline follow-back method (TLFB).
    B. Questions regarding average consumption practices.
    C. Prospective method.
    D. Retrospective diary method.
    E. Brown bag approach.

23.5 The timeline follow-back method is a commonly used technique for recording alcohol use in studies of addiction. A major limitation is

    A. It may overestimate use for less frequent users of alcohol.
    B. It is poorly correlated with reports from prospective diaries.
    C. It is less accurate when administered by an interviewer.
    D. The week being measured may not be representative of the person's usual drinking behavior.
    E. It may be administered more quickly than assessments of average alcohol frequency usage.

23.6 Which of the following is a long-term marker of alcohol use?

      A. Gamma-glutamyl transferase (GGT).
      B. Hematocrit.
      C. Blood urea nitrogen.
      D. Low-density lipoprotein level.
      E. Serum bilirubin.

23.7 In 1995 the U.S. Food and Drug Administration (FDA) approved the first medication in over 50 years for the treatment of alcohol dependence. Which of the following is the medication?

      A. Disulfiram.
      B. Naltrexone.
      C. Naloxone.
      D. Acamprosate.
      E. Bupropion.

C h a p t e r   2 4

Personality Disorders

Select the single best response for each question.

24.1 You are asked to evaluate a 75-year-old woman who was referred by her internist. She exhibits the following long-standing characteristics: sensitivity to rejection and chronic feelings of abandonment. You suspect that she has a personality disorder. Which of the following personality disorders is most likely?

   A. Avoidant.
   B. Borderline.
   C. Dependent.
   D. Paranoid.
   E. Schizoid.

24.2 Which of the following statements concerning personality disorders in seniors is *false*?

   A. The prevalence of personality disorders in older persons is generally twice the rate of personality disorders in younger persons in the general population.
   B. The single most common comorbid Axis I condition in seniors with personality disorders is depression.
   C. The prevalence of personality disorders in selected outpatient or inpatient samples of older persons can be as high as 25%–65%.
   D. The prevalence of personality disorders in the general population is estimated at 10%–15% of all ages.
   E. The prevalence of personality disorders in psychiatric settings is usually three to four times higher than in the community.

24.3 Both Erikson and Vaillant studied late-life development. All of the following statements concerning their work are true *except*

   A. Mature defenses were more consistently identified in Erickson's later developmental stages.
   B. Erikson proposed that the major developmental task of older age is to look back and seek meaning across the life span.
   C. An example of a mature and adaptive defense mechanism is suppression.
   D. Mature defenses are dependent upon education and social privilege.
   E. Mature defenses synthesize and attenuate conflicts.

24.4 You are asked by a colleague to evaluate an 80-year-old man for a possible personality disorder. You want to use a reliable and valid dimensional assessment tool that has proved useful as a screening tool in the elderly. Which of the following instruments would you select?

   A. Millon Clinical Multiaxial Inventory—III (MCMI-III).
   B. Personality Diagnostic Questionnaire (PDQ-IV).
   C. Schedule for Nonadaptive and Adaptive Personality.
   D. Wisconsin Personality Disorders Inventory.
   E. The Neuroticism, Extraversion, Openness Five Factor Model (NEO-FFM).

24.5 A 75-year-old woman whom you are called by a neurologist to evaluate was noted to have frontal lobe damage due to a motor vehicle accident. In evaluating her, you note many difficulties similar to which of the following personality disorders?

    A. Avoidant.
    B. Borderline.
    C. Dependent.
    D. Obsessive-compulsive.
    E. Schizotypal.

Chapter 25

Agitation and Suspiciousness

Select the single best response for each question.

25.1 Kraepelin used the term *paraphrenia* to describe older patients who today would be most likely diagnosed according to DSM-IV-TR as having

    A. Dementia.
    B. Delirium.
    C. Delusional disorder.
    D. Schizoaffective disorder.
    E. Bipolar I disorder.

25.2 You ask the resident with whom you are working to outline some common nonpharmacological strategies for reducing agitation in an elderly patient whom you are treating. She comes up with the list below. You feel that all are good strategies *except*

    A. Focusing the person's attention on the triggering event so they will gain more understanding.
    B. Breaking down complex tasks into one-step guided directions.
    C. Simplifying instructions.
    D. Allowing adequate rest.
    E. Providing pleasant distractions specific to the person.

25.3 There are a number of communication strategies that may reduce a person's agitation. Which of the following is an example of one of these strategies?

    A. Avoid eye contact.
    B. Use popular expressions such as "don't go there."
    C. Ask the patient if he or she remembers you.
    D. Listen and don't feel compelled to talk constantly.
    E. Inquire as to what the patient wants to do, such as "Do you want to go now?"

25.4 You are called to evaluate a patient with Parkinson's disease who has become psychotic and agitated. An especially effective agent is

    A. Haloperidol.
    B. Quetiapine.
    C. Lorazepam.
    D. Aripiprazole.
    E. Pimozide.

25.5 When a patient is exhibiting agitation on a regular basis and neuroleptics are required, what is a good medication strategy to follow?

    A. Administer high doses of medication to treat specific episodes.
    B. Avoid high-potency agents such as haloperidol.
    C. Sedate the patient as much as possible.
    D. Use benzodiazepines in combination with neuroleptics.
    E. Administer low doses on a regular basis.

Chapter 26

Psychopharmacology

Select the single best response for each question.

26.1 Data show that all available selective serotonin reuptake inhibitors (SSRIs) have similar efficacy and tolerability in the treatment of depression in older adults; however, experts favor which of the following agents?

    A. Fluvoxamine.
    B. Paroxetine.
    C. Escitalopram.
    D. Fluoxetine.
    E. Duloxetine.

26.2 Which of the SSRIs needs to be administered twice a day in the elderly?

    A. Fluvoxamine.
    B. Paroxetine.
    C. Sertraline.
    D. Citalopram.
    E. Fluoxetine.

26.3 SSRIs may produce all of the following adverse side effects *except*

    A. Increased risk of post-surgical bleeding.
    B. Extrapyramidal symptoms.
    C. Fragility fractures.
    D. Tachycardia.
    E. Gastrointestinal bleeding.

26.4 With regard to the newer, non-SSRI antidepressants, which of the following may be less safe than sertraline in a frail, elderly population?

    A. Bupropion.
    B. Duloxetine.
    C. Mirtazapine.
    D. Nefazodone.
    E. Venlafaxine.

26.5 Which of the following newer antidepressants should be avoided in psychotic patients or in agitated patients at risk for the development of psychiatric symptoms?

    A. Bupropion.
    B. Duloxetine.
    C. Mirtazapine.
    D. Nefazodone.
    E. Venlafaxine.

26.6 Which of the following antidepressants has been approved by the U.S. Food and Drug Administration (FDA) for the treatment of pain associated with diabetic neuropathy?

    A. Bupropion.
    B. Duloxetine.
    C. Mirtazapine.
    D. Nefazodone.
    E. Venlafaxine.

26.7 Concerns have been expressed about which of the following newer antidepressants' adverse effects on cognition and driving performance?

    A. Bupropion.
    B. Duloxetine.
    C. Mirtazapine.
    D. Nefazodone.
    E. Venlafaxine.

26.8 Which of the following agents has been reported to increase the incidence of hepatic toxicity?

    A. Bupropion.
    B. Duloxetine.
    C. Mirtazapine.
    D. Nefazodone.
    E. Venlafaxine.

26.9 In Great Britain, the National Institute of Clinical Excellence has recommended that which of the following agents should not be prescribed to patients with preexisting heart disease?

    A. Bupropion.
    B. Duloxetine.
    C. Mirtazapine.
    D. Nefazodone.
    E. Venlafaxine.

26.10 If a TCA is to be prescribed to an older patient, which of the following agents is preferred?

    A. Amitriptyline.
    B. Clomipramine.
    C. Desipramine.
    D. Doxepin.
    E. Imipramine.

26.11 Of the atypical antipsychotics currently available in the United States, which has the most published geriatric data for a variety of conditions?

    A. Aripiprazole.
    B. Olanzapine.
    C. Quetiapine.
    D. Risperidone.
    E. Ziprasidone.

26.12 On review of all evidence available in 2004, a consensus conference concluded that among the atypical antipsychotics, which of the following had the highest risk for diabetes, weight gain, and dyslipidemia?

A. Aripiprazole.
B. Olanzapine.
C. Quetiapine.
D. Risperidone.
E. Ziprasidone.

26.13 Data suggest that which of the following antipsychotic agents should be first-line for the treatment of psychosis in patients with Parkinson's disease or dementia with Lewy bodies?

A. Aripiprazole.
B. Olanzapine.
C. Quetiapine.
D. Risperidone.
E. Ziprasidone.

26.14 Which of the following side effects has been reported with valproate in as many as half of elderly patients?

A. Hand tremors.
B. Pancreatitis.
C. Elevation in liver enzymes.
D. Thrombocytopenia.
E. Transient elevations in blood ammonia levels.

26.15 Which of the following mood stabilizers is *not* associated with weight gain?

A. Valproate.
B. Lamotrigine.
C. Lithium.
D. Carbamazepine.
E. Oxcarbazepine.

26.16 If a benzodiazepine must be prescribed to an elderly person for treatment of sleep disturbance, which of the following is preferred?

A. Clonazepam.
B. Alprazolam.
C. Triazolam.
D. Oxazepam.
E. Lorazepam.

26.17 Which of the following approved drugs for the treatment of Alzheimer's disease is an uncompetitive antagonist with moderate affinity for N-methyl-D-aspartate (NMDA) receptors?

A. Donepezil.
B. Memantine.
C. Rivastigmine.
D. Galantamine.
E. Tacrine.

Chapter 27

Electroconvulsive Therapy

Select the single best response for each question.

27.1 Electroconvulsive therapy (ECT) has been demonstrated to have efficacy in testing a number of specific conditions or disorders. For which of the following has ECT ***not*** been shown to be efficacious?

   A. Severe nonmelancholic depression.
   B. Negative symptoms of schizophrenia.
   C. Acute mania.
   D. Bipolar depression.
   E. Catatonia.

27.2 ECT is a highly effective treatment for a number of neuropsychiatric conditions; however, some patients who receive ECT for depression will relapse within 1 year after treatment with ECT, even when treated with typical continuation or maintenance pharmacotherapy. What is the estimated relapse rate for depressed patients 1 year after ECT treatment and when continued on pharmacotherapy?

   A. 5%–10%.
   B. 15%–20%.
   C. 25%–30%.
   D. 40%–49%.
   E. 50%–60%.

27.3 Pharmacotherapy is usually indicated after a successful course of ECT unless one of certain specific conditions exists. All of the following are examples of these contraindicating conditions ***except***

   A. The patient has a preference for maintenance ECT.
   B. Maintenance pharmacotherapy has failed in the past.
   C. The patient is intolerant of medications.
   D. The patient has previously responded to maintenance ECT.
   E. The patient has a medical illness that precludes medication.

27.4 Objective and subjective memory side effects of ECT have been shown to be greater in degree and duration under which of the following conditions?

   A. Lower stimulus intensity.
   B. More time between treatments.
   C. Larger number of ECT treatments.
   D. Unilateral placement of electrodes.
   E. Lower dosages of barbiturate anesthetic.

27.5 Certain psychotropic medications should be avoided or maintained at the lowest possible levels during ECT treatment. Which of the following is one of these medications?

    A. Lithium.
    B. Haloperidol.
    C. Sertraline.
    D. Olanzapine.
    E. Desipramine.

Chapter 28

Nutrition and Physical Activity

Select the single best response for each question.

28.1 Adherence to the Mediterranean diet has been associated with a reduced risk for cognitive decline. Which of the following is a component of the Mediterranean diet?

    A. High intake of trans-unsaturated fats.
    B. No ethanol consumption.
    C. High intake of saturated fats.
    D. High intake of poly-unsaturated fats.
    E. Low intake of mono-unsaturated fats.

28.2 There are three major components of nutritional assessment: dietary, biochemical, and clinical. The most commonly used biochemical assessment is for one or more markers of protein status. Which of the following markers has a very short half-life of 2–4 hours and a relatively small body pool, making it very sensitive to nutritional changes?

    A. Albumin.
    B. Prealbumin.
    C. Insulin-like growth factor 1 (IGF-1).
    D. Insulin.
    E. Transthyretin.

28.3 Although most nutritional experts recommend that all older adults take a multivitamin/mineral supplement, specific nutrients have been associated with adverse outcomes. Excessive intake of which of the following nutrients can interfere with copper status and impair immune function?

    A. Vitamin A.
    B. Zinc.
    C. Vitamin E.
    D. Folic acid.
    E. Iron.

28.4 A panel composed of public health, behavioral science, epidemiology, exercise science, medicine, and gerontology experts released recommendations on physical activity in older adults. Which of the following were its recommendations for aerobic activities?

    A. Mild-intensity aerobic activity at least 10 minutes each day, 7 days a week.
    B. Moderate-intensity aerobic activity at least 10 minutes each day, 7 days a week.
    C. Moderate-intensity aerobic activity at least 20 minutes each day, 7 days a week.
    D. Moderate-intensity aerobic activity at least 30 minutes each day, 5 days a week.
    E. Maximal-intensity aerobic activity at least 30 minutes each day, 7 days a week.

28.5 A number of nutrients have been linked to depression. Cross-sectional studies have associated depression with low levels of one of the nutrients below; however, longitudinal studies have failed to find an association. Which nutrient do these findings refer to?

A. Pyridoxine (B_6).
B. Folate (B_9).
C. Cobalamin (B_{12}).
D. Omega-3 fatty acids.
E. Saturated fats.

Chapter 29

Individual and Group Psychotherapy

Select the single best response for each question.

29.1 In the first known randomized trial examining cognitive-behavioral therapy (CBT) as a medication augmentation therapy, more than 100 depressed older adults were assigned to three treatment approaches: CBT alone, medication alone, or combined CBT and medication. What were the major findings?

 A. CBT alone had the greatest improvement over 16–20 weeks of treatment.
 B. CBT alone was significantly better than medication alone.
 C. The combined CBT and medication group reported the greatest improvements over 16–20 weeks of treatment.
 D. Medication alone was significantly better than CBT alone.
 E. Medication alone had the greatest improvement over 16–20 weeks of treatment.

29.2 Which of the following is a manualized treatment focused on four components (grief, interpersonal disputes, role transitions, and interpersonal deficits) that are hypothesized to lead to or maintain depression?

 A. Social problem-solving therapy (PST).
 B. Interpersonal psychotherapy (IPT).
 C. Cognitive-behavioral therapy.
 D. Psychodynamic psychotherapy.
 E. Cognitive therapy.

29.3 Investigators have studied the effects of exercise on depression in older adults. In one study, supervised exercise therapy, medication alone, and combined exercise and medication were evaluated to determine their effectiveness in treating depression in older adults. What was one of the results of this study?

 A. Medication alone was superior to supervised exercise therapy or combined exercise and medication therapy.
 B. Supervised exercise therapy was superior to medication alone or combined exercise and medication therapy.
 C. Combined exercise and medication therapy was superior to either medication alone or supervised exercise therapy.
 D. Follow-up assessments at 10 months revealed lower rates of depression in the medication group than in the supervised exercise therapy group or the combined treatment group.
 E. There were no significant differences among treatment groups.

29.4 Among older adults, the most commonly diagnosed anxiety disorder (believed to be underdiagnosed in older adults) is

 A. Panic disorder.
 B. Acute stress disorder.
 C. Social phobia.
 D. Generalized anxiety disorder (GAD).
 E. Obsessive-compulsive disorder.

29.5 The rate of personality disorder among depressed older adult samples has been estimated to be

    A. 5%.
    B. 10%.
    C. 15%.
    D. 20%.
    E. 30%.

Chapter 30

Working With Families of Older Adults

Select the single best response for each question.

30.1 For psychiatrists and other mental health professionals working with families, there are a number of clinical reminders that may prove useful. Which of the following is one of those clinical reminders?

    A. The family is frequently the obstacle to effective care for the older member.
    B. Different perceptions and expectations of close and distant family members do not necessarily result in family conflict.
    C. Denial on the part of family members must be confronted.
    D. A family caregiver's awareness of an available service invariably leads to appropriate use of that service.
    E. A primary caregiver at home is efficient and preferred.

30.2 Clinical goals for psychiatrists and other mental health professionals working with families of older adults will vary depending on presenting problems and family resources. However, some common goals are applicable to most families. All of the following are examples of these common clinical goals *except*

    A. To address safety issues.
    B. To help family members care for their elder member without needing outside help.
    C. To mobilize secondary family support.
    D. To facilitate appropriate decision making at care transitions.
    E. To normalize variability.

30.3 Families have certain expectations of psychiatrists. Which of the following is one of these expectations?

    A. Families want action from psychiatrists and not listening.
    B. Psychiatrists should not ask what else is going on in the family's lives since they already have much to deal with.
    C. Families appreciate general suggestions from psychiatrists to take care of themselves.
    D. Families look to psychiatrists for support in making certain decisions.
    E. Psychiatrists should discourage family members from expressing their feelings.

30.4 It is important for the psychiatrist to assess the family of an older adult. All of the following are examples of effective assessment *except*

    A. Asking about other family commitments.
    B. Carefully assessing cultural expectations.
    C. Avoiding asking about previous and current help from family members.
    D. Assessing family strengths, skills, and goals.
    E. Asking the family to describe a typical day.

30.5   There are a number of key messages that psychiatrists should convey to family caregivers over time. Which of the following is one of these messages?

    A. You can only do what is best at the time. Doubts will occur.
    B. Avoid expressing your honest feelings to anyone since your conversation may get back to the older adult.
    C. Try not to compromise among competing needs, loyalties, or commitments. Make firm commitments.
    D. Save your time and energy to celebrate major, not minor, successes.
    E. The older adult may often be unhappy with what you have done.

Chapter 31

Clinical Psychiatry in the Nursing Home

Select the single best response for each question.

31.1 Epidemiological studies during the 1980s and 1990s reported prevalence rates for psychiatric disorders among nursing home residents. On the basis of psychiatric interviews of nursing home patients in randomly selected samples, investigators reported rates for psychiatric disorders in which of the following ranges?

   A. 50%–55%.
   B. 60%–65%.
   C. 70%–75%.
   D. 80%–85%.
   E. 90%–95%.

31.2 Dementia is the most common psychiatric disorder in nursing home patients. What is the second most common psychiatric disorder?

   A. Generalized anxiety disorder.
   B. Depression.
   C. Schizophrenia.
   D. Bipolar disorder.
   E. Alcoholism.

31.3 A number of nonpharmacological interventions have proven to be effective in reducing agitation in nursing home patients. Which of the following has **not** been shown to be effective in reducing agitation?

   A. Daytime physical activity combined with a nighttime program to decrease noise and sleep-disruptive nursing care practices.
   B. Activities matched to skills and interest of patients.
   C. Bright light therapy.
   D. Individualized modification in the physical environment.
   E. Individualized consultation for staff nurses about the management of patients with dementia.

31.4 Efficacy of some of the atypical antipsychotic agents for the treatment of psychotic symptoms and agitated behavior in nursing home residents without dementia has been demonstrated in several multicenter randomized, double-blind, placebo-controlled clinical trials. Which of the following agents has **not** been studied in this manner?

   A. Aripiprazole.
   B. Olanzapine.
   C. Quetiapine.
   D. Risperidone.
   E. Ziprasidone.

31.5 Analyses of safety data from randomized, controlled studies of atypical antipsychotic drugs in elderly patients with dementia revealed significantly increased risks of cerebrovascular adverse events and mortality. Which of the following agents had the highest rate of cerebrovascular adverse events?

A. Aripiprazole.
B. Olanzapine.
C. Quetiapine.
D. Risperidone.
E. Ziprasidone.

31.6 Although selective serotonin reuptake inhibitors (SSRIs) generally are well tolerated by frail elderly nursing home patients, this class of antidepressants has been associated with which of the following adverse events?

A. Falls.
B. Strokes.
C. Diabetes.
D. Delirium.
E. Hypertension.

31.7 Regulations promulgated by the Health Care Financing Administration require that nursing home residents not receive unnecessary drugs. An unnecessary drug is defined by all of the following *except*

A. Excessive duration.
B. Inadequate dose.
C. Without adequate monitoring.
D. Without adequate indications.
E. In the presence of adverse consequences.

Chapter 32

The Continuum of Caring in the Long Term

Movement Toward the Community

Select the single best response for each question.

32.1 In the U.S. population, disability that results in institutional care has been

A. Increasing at the rate of about 1% a year.
B. Increasing at the rate of about 5% a year.
C. Remaining constant.
D. Decreasing at the rate of about 1% a year.
E. Decreasing at the rate of about 5% a year.

32.2 The most notable example of federal policy innovation in long-term care is the modification of Medicaid under the Reagan administration's home- and community-based care (HCBS) waivers. This provision

A. Excluded nursing homes from receiving Medicaid except under special circumstances.
B. Reduced funding for nursing homes.
C. Enabled states to seek waivers for home- and community-based options for older and disabled beneficiaries who normally would require nursing care.
D. Enabled states to seek waivers creating acute inpatient units for short stays for the older and disabled.
E. Excluded federal reimbursement for patients with psychiatric disorders who were admitted to nursing homes.

32.3 Hospice care is designed to achieve a number of goals. Which of the following is *not* one of these goals?

A. Maximize a sense of self-efficacy in individuals.
B. Manage a terminal patient's final transition in a minimally medical environment.
C. Provide social and emotional support to the patient.
D. Create a sense of collective self-efficacy for families.
E. Provide access to the latest technological innovations.

32.4 Consumer-directed care has been slower to develop among older adults primarily because of

A. Lack of financial support for innovative alternatives.
B. Concerns about whether older persons are capable.
C. Concerns over increased possible costs of alternative services.
D. Questions about the role of federal and state agencies.
E. Lack of consensus as to what needs to be done.

32.5 The basic concepts of the distinctive philosophy of assisted-living housing include all of the following *except*

    A. Allowing families to have more decision-making authority.
    B. Matching services with individual need.
    C. Offering a private, self-contained space of one's own.
    D. Sharing responsibility for care among residents, family, and staff.
    E. Enhancing the availability to residents of information for informed choice.

32.6 In health services research on mental health in the United States, the major issue that is discussed often and early is

    A. Access concerns.
    B. The role of primary care physicians.
    C. Making an accurate diagnosis.
    D. Costs.
    E. Evidence-based practices.

Chapter 33

Legal, Ethical, and Policy Issues

Select the single best response for each question.

33.1 The Omnibus Budget Reconciliation Act of 1987 (OBRA-87) made a number of changes to how Medicare covered outpatient psychiatric services. Which of the following changes occurred as a result of this legislation?

A. Allowed licensed clinical psychologists to bill Medicare for mental health services.
B. Changed the copayment for psychotherapy services from 50% to 20%.
C. Raised the cap for psychiatry reimbursement to $2,200.
D. Eliminated the cap on outpatient mental health services.
E. Allowed licensed certified social workers to bill Medicare for mental health services.

33.2 Between the years of 1990 and 2000, a number of changes occurred in the demographic characteristics of veterans receiving mental health services from the Department of Veterans Affairs (VA). Which of the following was one of these changes?

A. There was a fourfold decrease in the number of veterans ages 75–84 who received mental health services.
B. The most rapid increase in demand for services was from younger veterans (ages 35–44).
C. Fewer than 5 million veterans are over age 65.
D. The number of veterans in the 45- to 54-year-old age group who received mental health services more than tripled.
E. The number of Vietnam-era veterans receiving mental health services is declining each year.

33.3 Numerous reviews and professional organizations' position statements have set forth guidelines for what constitutes good care at the end of life. Some common fundamentals have emerged. All of the following are examples of these fundamentals *except*

A. Education and training of both professional and informal caregivers.
B. Support of family and caregivers before and after the death of the patient.
C. Maximizing quality of life.
D. Removal of regulatory barriers to access care.
E. Delay advance planning and preparation for death and focus on the here and now.

33.4 A variety of techniques are available to psychiatrists to improve the quality of communication among patients, families, and health care professionals. Which of the following is *not* one of these techniques?

A. Avoid clarifying vague terms so as not to make the patient more anxious.
B. Identify a proxy decision maker.
C. Identify patient concerns about the future.
D. Learn the patient's understanding about potential outcomes.
E. Learn about the patient's concept of quality of life.

33.5 What is it called when a person makes a decision for a patient on the basis of what the patient's wishes would be were the patient capable of making the decision?

    A. Living will.
    B. Substituted judgment.
    C. Power of attorney.
    D. Guardianship.
    E. Durable power of attorney.

Chapter 34

The Past and Future of Geriatric Psychiatry

Select the single best response for each question.

34.1 Geriatric psychiatry faces special problems in obtaining referrals. Which is an example of one of these problems?

    A. Inadequate training of geriatric psychiatrists to handle the referral questions.
    B. Lack of need for specialized geriatric services.
    C. Discouragement of referrals by managed care systems.
    D. Improved training of primary care physicians to manage most problems.
    E. Lack of demonstrated cost-effectiveness.

34.2 What is the major difficulty facing geriatric psychiatry fellowship training programs?

    A. Prejudices about aging from younger physicians.
    B. Lack of quality training programs.
    C. Inadequate knowledge base for the field of geriatric psychiatry.
    D. Low reimbursement for clinical services.
    E. No certification examination like child psychiatry.

34.3 You admit one of your geriatric patients, who is covered by Medicare, to an inpatient psychiatric unit in the general hospital where you have admission privileges. The spouse asks you what Medicare will cover in terms of expenses. Which of the following is correct?

    A. Medicare has a 190-day lifetime psychiatric hospitalization limit for patients admitted to psychiatric units in general hospitals.
    B. There will be a one-time deductible of $768 for the first 60 days.
    C. Medicare does not pay after day 60 of a single hospitalization.
    D. There will be a daily co-pay for the first 60 days.
    E. Medicare does not reimburse patients for inpatient stays at freestanding psychiatric hospitals.

34.4 Criteria that have been suggested as markers of successful aging include all of the following *except*

    A. Overall intelligence (IQ).
    B. Resiliency.
    C. Personal control.
    D. Life satisfaction.
    E. Adaptability.

34.5 Wisdom in successful aging has been defined by Baltes (1993). Which elements of such wisdom does Baltes describe as "recognizing that no perfect solution exists"?

    A. Factual knowledge.
    B. Procedural knowledge.
    C. Lifespan contextualization.
    D. Value relativism.
    E. Acceptance of uncertainty.

Chapter 1

The Myth, History, and Science of Aging

Select the single best response for each question.

1.1   A number of scientists have studied human tissues and cells to investigate the process of aging. Which of the following investigators became convinced that some human cells grown in culture were immortal?

    A. Hayflick and Moorhead.

    B. Medvedev.

    C. Carrel.

    D. Lepeshinskaya.

    E. Bacon.

The correct response is option C.

Alexis Carrel (1873–1944), a surgeon, devoted much work to wound healing. This interest in wound healing led him to an interest in growing tissues outside the body. For his surgical contributions, he won the 1912 Nobel Prize for physiology and medicine. He subsequently developed his studies in tissue culture, and on the basis of some of his own apparent successes, he became convinced that some human cells grown in culture were immortal. This claim of possible cell immortality was reported by Carrel and Ebeling beginning in 1912. Despite numerous objections to his work, Carrel was very persuasive, and his belief was widely accepted.

Hayflick and Moorhead (1961) first described the finite replicative capacity of cultured normal human fibroblasts and interpreted this phenomenon as aging at the cellular level. They reported that even when normal human embryonic cells were grown under the most favorable conditions, death was inevitable after about 50 population doublings. Thus, the death of the cell line was an inherent property of the cells themselves.

Around 1949, Lepeshinskaya began to advocate the use of soda baths to prolong life and restore vigor. This approach quickly moved to the drinking of soda water and finally to the introduction of soda into the body by enema. Apparently the latter two techniques were used as alternatives for those who were unable to take frequent soda baths. Lepeshinskaya also claimed that she could make living matter from nonliving material, a vivid example of how vulnerable geriatrics is to the practice of pseudoscience.

Zhores Medvedev, a Russian scientist, made many contributions to the study of biological aging, including the redundant theory of aging (i.e., the amount of DNA reserve within the genome that can be called on to maintain vital function plays an important role in determining life span; Busse 1983). Roger Bacon (ca. 1214–ca. 1292) promoted his belief that the life span of his day, which usually was not more than 45–50 years, could be tripled. His reasoning was in part based on the long life spans of Methuselah and Noah: if life spans had once been that long and then had shortened, some reversal must be possible. **(p. 4)**

1.2   A number of theories of aging have been proposed by various investigators. Which one of the following types of theories holds that aging is the result of sequential switching on and off of certain genes, and that defects develop during this switching on and off?

    A. Error theories.
    B. Somatic mutation theories.
    C. Cellular-based theories.
    D. Program theories.
    E. Exhaustion theories.

The correct response is option D.

Program theories hold that aging is the result of sequential switching on and off of certain genes. Defects develop during this switching on and off, and these defects are manifested by senescence.

Those who subscribe to error theories maintain that aging is the result of wear-and-tear processes; these theorists hold that in many mechanisms, important parts wear out and cannot be replaced or repaired. Included among the error theories is the somatic mutation theory, whose proponents maintain that, with increasing age, genetic mutations occur and accumulate, causing cells to deteriorate and malfunction.

The cellular-based theories are those that emphasize the importance of the inherent limited potential proliferation of cells. These theories are consistent with the fact that animals have decreased cellularity in several organs as aging advances.

One early biological explanation of aging rested on the assumption that a living organism contains a fixed store of energy not unlike that contained within a coiled watch spring. When the spring of the watch is unwound, life ends. This is a type of exhaustion theory. **(pp. 7–8)**

1.3   Processes of aging that are associated with random changes, such as cell loss or mutation, are part of which of the following theories?

    A. Stochastic theory.
    B. The master clock.
    C. Deliberate biological programming.
    D. The telomere theory.
    E. The free radical theory.

The correct response is option A.

Processes of aging that are associated with random changes, such as cell loss or mutation, are often termed *stochastic* processes. Stochastic implies "a process or a series of events for which the estimate of the probability of certain outcomes approaches the true possibility as the number of events increases" (Busse 1977, p. 16). The atomic scientist Leo Szilard advanced a stochastic theory based on what he termed a "hit." A hit is not solely the result of radiation but rather can be considered any event that alters a chromosome.

The hypothalamus is said to be the location of the "master clock." Age changes within the hypothalamus play a particularly important role in losses of homeostatic mechanisms in the body. Cell loss, an event that is common in late life, occurs within clusters of cells in the hypothalamus. The disappearance of a few critical cells in the hypothalamus may have far-reaching consequences.

The theory of deliberate biological programming holds that within a normal cell are stored the memory and the capability of determining the life of a cell. This theory is consistent with the research and conclusions of Hayflick (1965). The memory and capacity to terminate life are found in all normal human diploid cells. In mixoploid or cancer cells, this memory or capacity apparently is destroyed, and the cells can duplicate indefinitely.

A variant of the deliberate biological programming theory and also of the genetic theories is the telomere theory. DNA damage is the centerpiece of many theories of aging. Telomere shortening has been described to be associated with DNA damage (Ahmed and Tollefsbol 2001). Located at the ends of eukaryotic chromosomes, telomeres are specialized DNA sequences that maintain the length of chromosomes. When they are lost, DNA damages results.

A free radical is a chemical molecule or compound that has an odd number of electrons (an unpaired electron) and is highly reactive, in contrast to most chemical compounds, which have an even number of electrons and are stable. Often considered molecular fragments, free radicals are highly reactive and destructive, but they are produced by normal metabolic processes and are ubiquitous in living substances. They can also be produced by ionizing radiation, ozone, and chemical toxins such as insecticides. The oxygen free radical, superoxide, is an important agent of oxygen toxicity and the aging process. (pp. 8–9)

1.4   There are a number of genetic syndromes that are linked with premature aging. Although all of these are quite rare, one is characterized by dwarfism, physical immaturity, pseudosenility, and hypermetabolism. The affected individuals usually die in their mid-teens of coronary heart disease. Which of the following is this disorder?

     A. Werner's syndrome.
     B. Hutchinson-Gilford syndrome.
     C. Down syndrome.
     D. Laurence-Seip syndrome.
     E. Cockayne's syndrome.

The correct response is option B.

The early-onset Hutchinson-Gilford syndrome is characterized by dwarfism, physical immaturity, and pseudosenility. Individuals with this syndrome have a peculiar form of hypermetabolism, and they generally die during their mid-teens of coronary heart disease. Hutchinson-Gilford syndrome affects both sexes and has been described in white, black, and Asian races. The affected individuals look like very old, wizened, small humans with distorted features. Some of the features that are commonly associated with aging, including tumors, cataracts, and osteoporosis, are not increased in Hutchinson-Gilford syndrome. A biochemical defect found in patients with Hutchinson-Gilford syndrome or Werner's syndrome is decreased excretion of urinary hyaluronic acid.

The appearance of an individual affected by Werner's syndrome is indeed striking because the initial impression is that the person is very old. As the disease develops, affected individuals look 20–30 years older than their actual years, and their life span is shortened. Because the disease usually appears before growth is completed, patients with this syndrome frequently have thin limbs and typically are of smaller stature and are less developed than would be expected. Their face develops a tightly drawn, pinched expression. Pseudoexophthalmos (bulging eyes), a beak nose, protuberant teeth, and a recessive chin are characteristic features. Cataracts develop early, and, in addition to hypogonadism, individuals are likely to have diabetes. Not infrequently, they develop cancer, which contributes to their shortened life expectancy. Martin (1978) reviewed a long list of human genetic conditions to select out those in which physical and physiological changes usually were associated with senescence. He identified the 10 genetic disorders that had the highest number of senescent features and thus that were considered to be associated with the aging process: Down syndrome, Werner's syndrome, Cockayne's syndrome, progeria, ataxia-telangiectasia, Lawrence-Seip syndrome, cervical lipodysplasia, Klinefelter's syndrome, Turner's syndrome, and myotonic dystrophy.

The progerias are syndromes that are linked with premature aging. The presence of these disorders does, to a limited extent, provide an opportunity to study accelerated bodily changes that resemble those attributable to aging. Although all of these syndromes are quite rare, two have received particular attention: Hutchinson-Gilford syndrome (Hastings 1904; Hutchinson 1886) and Werner's syndrome. Werner's syndrome is a later-onset type of progeria. Werner described the condition in siblings, two brothers and two sisters, between ages 36 and 40 years, whose parents, grandparents, and one sister were healthy. Because Werner's syndrome differs from normal aging in several respects, Martin (1985) classified this condition as a "segmental progeroid syndrome." **(pp. 10–11)**

1.5   There are a number of sex differences in longevity. Which of the following statements concerning men and women is *false*?

   A. Before 1900, in those nations where data are available, there were slightly more older men than older women.
   B. In 2007, the life expectancy for females was 7 years longer than for males in Japan.
   C. The single most important cause of higher mortality in males than females is an increased incidence of cigarette smoking in males.
   D. In non-industrial societies, women are more vulnerable to infectious diseases than men, leading to higher mortality rates.
   E. In the United States there are equal numbers of males and females born.

The correct response is option E.

Contrary to the reasonable expectation of the equal balance in males and females at birth, there are in the United States approximately 106–110 white males born for every 100 white females and approximately 104 black males born for every 100 black females.

In countries where data are available, there seemed to be slightly more older men than older women before 1900. After the turn of the century, this situation gradually changed, and by 1940 the situation had reversed itself. Thereafter, the preponderance of older women increased rapidly. In 2003, in the population older than 65 years, the sex ratio was 58% women to 42% men.

The female in the more developed nations has a life expectancy of 8 or more years beyond that of the male. In 1978, France had the most extreme female–male differences for life expectancy at birth: 8.21 years. In Japan this female–male difference is increasing: in 2007 the life expectancy in Japan was 86 years for females and 79 years for males.

Waldron (1986) noted that in contemporary industrial societies, the single most important cause of higher mortality for males has been a greater incidence of cigarette smoking among men. Other sex differences in mortality are related to behaviors that contribute to the males' higher mortality. Such behaviors include heavier alcohol consumption and employment in hazardous occupations.

In nonindustrial societies, women are more vulnerable to infectious diseases. This may be related to less adequate nutrition and health care for women. **(pp. 11–12)**

1.6   A number of social theories of aging have been proposed. Proponents of one theoretical approach maintain that older people tend to behave according to a pattern that has been established before late life. Which theory does this describe?

   A. The disengagement theory.
   B. The activity theory.
   C. The continuity theory.
   D. The age stratification theory.
   E. The life events and stress theory.

The correct response is option C.

The *continuity approach* is something of a compromise position between the disengagement and activity theories (Neugarten 1964). Proponents of the continuity approach maintain that older people tend to behave according to a pattern that has been established before late life. At times the person may disengage and at other times remain active. It is also apparent that some elderly people will drop one type of activity only to replace it with something that is more suitable to their health status and environment.

Disengagement theory states that aging invariably causes physical, psychological, and social disengagement (Cumming and Henry 1961). Physical disengagement is attributable to a decline in physical energy, a decline in strength, and the slowing of responses. Psychological disengagement refers to the withdrawal of concern from a rather diffuse interest in many people to a focus on those who are directly related to the individual.

Shortly after the appearance of the disengagement theory, the *activity theory* was proposed (Havighurst 1963). This theory holds that activity positively affects health, happiness, and longevity and that remaining active is good for both the aging individual and society.

Age stratification is really a model of life span development but obviously includes late life as a part of the conceptualization. According to Palmore (1981), age stratification conceptualizes society as being composed of different age groups with different roles and different expectations. Each age group must move up through time while responding to changes in environment. Age stratification focuses on distinguishing between age, period, and cohort effects.

The *life events and stress theory* holds that those major events usually associated with advancing age are particularly important to health and well-being in late life. A study using this approach must distinguish events that may be welcomed or resisted from those that do not affect all people in a similar manner. Some people resist retirement, whereas others welcome it. Some are unhappy in retirement, whereas others see it as an opportunity to attain life satisfactions. (p. 14)

References

Ahmed A, Tollefsbol T: Telomeres and telomerase: basic science implications for aging. J Am Geriatr Soc 49:1105–1109, 2001

Busse EW: Theories of aging, in Behavior and Adaptation in Late Life, 2nd Edition. Edited by Busse EW, Pfeiffer E. Boston, MA, Little, Brown, 1977, pp 11–32

Busse EW: Biologic and psychosocial bases of behavioral changes in aging, in Psychiatry Update: The American Psychiatric Association Annual Review, Vol 2. Edited by Grinspoon L. Washington, DC, American Psychiatric Press, 1983, pp 96–106

Cumming E, Henry W: Growing Old. New York, Basic Books, 1961

Havighurst R: Successful aging, in Processes of Aging. Edited by Williams R, Tibbitts C, Donahue W. New York, Atherton Press, 1963, pp 81–90

Hayflick L: The limited in vitro lifetime of human diploid cell strains. Exp Cell Res 37:614–616, 1965

Hayflick L, Moorhead PS: The serial cultivation of human diploid cell strains. Exp Cell Res 25:585–621, 1961

Hastings G: Progeria: a form of senilism. Practitioner 73:188–217, 1904

Hutchinson J: Case of congenital absence of hair and mammary glands with atrophic condition of the skin and its appendages. Lancet 1:473–477, 1886

Martin GM: Genetic syndromes in man with potential relevance to the pathobiology of aging: genetics of aging. Birth Defects Orig Artic Ser 14:5–39, 1978

Martin GM: Genetics and aging: the Werner syndrome as a segmental progeroid syndrome, in Werner's Syndrome and Human Aging (Advances in Experimental Medicine and Biology, Vol 190). Edited by Salk D, Fujiwara Y, Martin GM. New York, Plenum, 1985, pp 161–170

Neugarten B: Personality in Middle and Later Life. New York, Atherton Press, 1964

Palmore E: Social Patterns in Normal Aging: Findings From the Duke Longitudinal Study. Durham, NC, Duke University Press, 1981

Waldron I: What do we know about causes of sex differences in mortality: a review of the literature. Population Bulletin of the United Nations 18:59–76, 1986

Werner O: [Cataract in connection with scleroderma] (in German). Doctoral dissertation, Ophthalmological Clinic, Kiel, Germany, 1904

Chapter 2

Demography and Epidemiology of Psychiatric Disorders in Late Life

Select the single best response for each question.

2.1 Which of the following demographic statistics concerning older adults is *true*?

   A. In 2000, approximately 12.3 million persons in the United States were age 65 or older.
   B. In 2000, the number of "oldest old" or persons age 85 or older was 2.1 million.
   C. Nursing home residence has increased in recent years.
   D. The life expectancy in the United States for women has increased from 48.3 years in 1900 to 80.4 years in 2004.
   E. The percentage of men 70 or older in the labor force has increased from 20.8% in 1903 to 32.8% in 2003.

The correct response is option D.

In 1900, life expectancy in the United States was 48.3 years for females and 46.3 years for males, whereas in 2004, the life expectancy at birth was 80.4 years for females and 75.2 years for males. In 2004, a 65-year-old could expect to live an average of 18.7 more years, and a 75-year-old could expect to live 11.9 additional years (National Center for Health Statistics 2006).

In 2000, approximately 35 million persons ages 65 years or older lived in the United States, accounting for more than 12% of the population. Over the last century, the number of persons in this age group steadily increased, from 3.1 million in 1900 and 12.3 million in 1950 to the current estimate. Even more astounding, in 2000, the number of "oldest old," or persons age 85 years or older, was 4.2 million and was projected to reach 20.9 million by 2050 (Federal Interagency Forum on Aging-Related Statistics 2006).

Although nursing home residence has declined in recent years, the rate among those age 65 years or older in 1999 was 43.3 per 1,000, and the rate for those age 85 or older was 182.5 per 1,000 (Federal Interagency Forum on Aging-Related Statistics 2006).

The percentage of older adults in the labor force—those who are either working or looking for work—has changed over the last four decades. The percentage of men ages 65–69 years in the labor force declined from 1963 (40.9%) to 1983 (26.1%) and then increased to 32.8% by 2003. The percentage of men age 70 years or older in the labor force declined from 20.8% in 1963 to 12.3% in 2003. **(pp. 19–20)**

2.2 Diagnostic categories that approximate true disease processes should have several characteristics. Which of the following is *not* one of these characteristics?

   A. A category should predict the outcome of a disorder.
   B. A category should reflect underlying biological reality.
   C. The classification scheme should identify persons who would not be responsive to a specific therapeutic intervention.
   D. Laboratory studies should eventually validate a diagnostic category.
   E. A category should be distinguished on the basis of patterns of symptomatology.

The correct response is option C.

Diagnostic categories that approximate true disease processes have several characteristics, including the following (Weissman and Klerman 1978): 1) a category should be distinguished on the basis of patterns of symptomatology (e.g., the clustering of symptoms in vascular depression) (Alexopoulos et al. 1997); 2) a category should predict the outcome of a disorder (e.g., Alzheimer's disease should predict a steady decline in cognitive functioning) (Shoghi-Jadid et al. 2002); 3) a category should reflect underlying biological reality, confirmed by family and genetic studies (e.g., Alzheimer's disease) (Roses 1994); 4) laboratory studies should eventually validate a diagnostic category (e.g., the use of specific imaging studies to diagnose Alzheimer's disease) (Roses 1997); 5) the classification scheme should identify persons who may respond to a specific therapeutic intervention, such as a particular form of psychotherapy or a specific group of medications (e.g., the use of combined pharmacotherapy and interpersonal psychotherapy to treat late-life depression) (Reynolds et al. 1999). **(p. 21)**

2.3   One of the landmark studies of the prevalence of psychiatric disorders in the United States was the Epidemiologic Catchment Area (ECA) survey. Which of the following statements concerning the ECA is *true*?

   A. The ECA sought to determine the prevalence of specific psychiatric disorders in community, but not institutional settings.
   B. Data were collected in three communities.
   C. The most prevalent disorder in individuals 65 or older was depressive disorder.
   D. The diagnoses were based on DSM-IV criteria.
   E. A total of 12.3% of those 65 or older met criteria for one or more psychiatric disorders in the month prior to the interview.

The correct response is option E.

One of the landmark studies of the prevalence of psychiatric disorders in the United States was the ECA survey conducted more than two decades ago. The National Institute of Mental Health established the ECA program to determine the prevalence of specific psychiatric disorders in both community and institutional populations (Regier et al. 1984). Data were collected in five communities, and the DIS was used to identify persons who met criteria for specific disorders. DIS diagnoses were based on DSM-III criteria (American Psychiatric Association 1980), the nomenclature in effect at the time the data were collected. More than 18,000 persons were interviewed in the ECA study, including 5,702 persons who were age 65 or older. All disorders, with the exception of cognitive impairment, were more prevalent in younger or middle-aged adults than in older adults. Of those age 65 or older, 12.3% (13.6% of the women and 10.5% of the men) met criteria for one or more psychiatric disorders in the month prior to the interview. The two most prevalent disorders in this age group were any anxiety disorder (5.5%) and severe cognitive impairment (4.9%) (Regier et al. 1988). **(p. 23)**

2.4   The prevalence of psychiatric disorders in community populations of older adults (age 55 or older) is relatively consistent across most disorders. Which of the following prevalence rates is *false*?

   A. The prevalence rate of major depression generally ranged from 1%–3%.
   B. The prevalence of individual disorders was highest for panic disorder (3%–10%).
   C. The prevalence of any anxiety disorder in the ECA studies was 5.5%.
   D. The prevalence of anxiety disorders is higher than that of major depression.
   E. The prevalence of alcohol abuse/dependence was low (0.1%–1.5%).

The correct response is option B.

TABLE 2–1. Prevalence of selected psychiatric disorders in community populations of older adults

Authors	Sample	N	Age	Disorder	Period	Prevalence
Hasin et al. 2007	National Epidemiologic Survey on Alcoholism and Related Conditions	8,205 65+ (from total U.S. representative sample of 43,093)	65+	Alcohol use disorder	12 months	1.5%
					Lifetime	16.1%
Hasin et al. 2005	"	"	"	Major depression	12 months	2.7%
					Lifetime	8.2%
Grant et al. 2006	"	"	"	Panic disorder	12 months	0.8%
					Lifetime	2.8%
Grant et al. 2005a	"	"	"	Social anxiety disorder	12 months	1.6%
					Lifetime	3.0%
Grant et al. 2005b	"	"	"	Generalized anxiety	12 months	1.0%
					Lifetime	2.6%
Stinson et al. 2007	"	"	"	Specific phobia	12 months	7.5%
Trollor et al. 2007	Australian National Mental Health and Well-Being Survey	1,792	65+	Major depression	1 month	1.2%
				Dysthymia		0.2%
				Panic disorder/agoraphobia		0.3%
				Social phobia		0.1%
				Generalized anxiety disorder		0.8%
				Posttraumatic stress disorder		0.2%
				Alcohol abuse/dependence		0.3%
Kessler et al. 2005	National Comorbidity Survey Replication	1,837 60+ (from total U.S. representative sample of 9,282)	60+	Major depression	Lifetime	10.6%
				Dysthymia		1.3%
				Panic disorder		2.0%
				Agoraphobia without panic		1.0%
				Specific phobia		7.5%
				Social phobia		6.6%
				Generalized anxiety disorder		3.6%
				Posttraumatic stress disorder		2.5%
				Obsessive-compulsive disorder		0.7%
				Alcohol abuse		6.2%
				Alcohol dependence		2.2%
Ritchie et al. 2004	Montpelier district of France	1,873	65+	Anxiety disorders	Current	14.2%
				Phobia		10.7%
				Major depression		3.0%
				Psychosis		1.7%
ESEMeD/MHEDEA 2000 Investigators 2004	European Study of the Epidemiology of Mental Disorders (ESEMeD)	4,401 age 65+ (from total sample of 21,425)	65+	Any mood disorder	12 months	3.2%
				Any anxiety disorder		3.6%
				Any alcohol disorder		0.1%

TABLE 2–1. Prevalence of selected psychiatric disorders in community populations of older adults *(continued)*

Authors	Sample	N	Age	Disorder	Period	Prevalence
Steffens et al. 2000	Cache County (UT) study	4,559	65+	Major depression	Current	4.4% female 2.7% male
Beekman et al. 1995	LASA	3,056	55–85	Major depression	Current	2.0%
Blazer et al. 1991b	Durham, North Carolina, ECA	784	65+	Generalized anxiety disorder		2.2%
Lindesay et al. 1989	Guy's/Age Concern Survey	890	65+	Phobic disorder	Current	10.0%
Bland et al. 1988	Edmonton, AB, Canada	358	65+	Major depression	Current	1.2%
				Phobic disorder		3.0%
				Panic disorder		0.3%
Regier et al. 1988	ECA in five U.S. communities	5,702 age 65+ (from total sample of 18,571)	65+	Major depression	1 month	0.7%
				Dysthymia		1.8%
				Any anxiety disorder		5.5%
				Phobic disorder		4.8%
				Schizophrenia		0.1%
				Alcohol abuse/dependence		0.9%
Copeland et al. 1987	Liverpool, England	1,070	65+	Depressive neurosis	Current	8.3%
				Depressive psychosis		2.9%

Note. ECA = Epidemiologic Catchment Area; LASA = Longitudinal Aging Studies Amsterdam.

2.4 *(continued)*

As shown in Table 2–1, the prevalence of individual disorders is highest for phobic disorders (3%–10%) and lowest for panic disorder (<1%). The current prevalence of major depression ranges from 0.7% reported from the ECA (Regier et al. 1988) to 3% reported from a survey in France (Ritchie et al. 2004), and somewhat higher in the Cache County (Utah) survey (Steffens et al. 2000). Overall, the findings are fairly consistent, with prevalence estimates from the rest of the studies presented falling within that range of 1%–3%. The prevalence is higher in older females than males (Regier et al. 1988; Steffens et al. 2000).

The prevalence of any anxiety disorder among adults age 65 or older in the ECA studies was 5.5%, with a higher prevalence in females (6.8%) than in males (3.6%) (Regier et al.1988).

The current prevalence of anxiety disorders is higher than that of major depression, and the estimates depend in part on whether specific phobia is included.

The prevalence of alcohol abuse/dependence was low (0.1%–1.5%) (Regier et al. 1988; Trollor et al. 2007). (pp. 28–30)

2.5   Which of the following statements concerning psychiatric disorders in older adults is **true**?

   A. Psychiatric disorders are found at a higher prevalence among the elderly than at other stages of the life cycle.
   B. DSM-IV-TR provides age-specific categories for elderly persons, similar to children.
   C. The prevalence of major depression in nursing homes or long-term care facilities (1%–3%) is no different from prevalence in community samples of older adults.
   D. Suicide mortality is positively correlated with age.
   E. Older women are less likely to die from suicide than young women.

The correct response is option D.

Suicide mortality is positively correlated with age. Suicide mortality worldwide in 2000 was more than twice as high for older men (50.0 per 100,000 men age 75 years or older) as for young men (22.0 per 100,000 men ages 15–24 years), according to pooled data from the World Health Organization (2000).

   Overall, psychiatric disorders are found at a lower prevalence among elderly people than in people at other stages of the life cycle. In the ECA, the 1-month prevalence of any Diagnostic Interview Schedule disorder (including cognitive impairment) was 16.9% in those ages 18–24 years, 17.3% in those ages 25–44 years, 13.3% in those ages 45–64 years, and 12.3% in those age 65 years or older (Regier et al. 1988).

   DSM-IV-TR provides age-specific categories for children but not for elderly persons. Clinicians who work with older adults, however, have often commented that depression may be masked in late life by symptoms of poor physical health or pseudodementia. Yet there is no compelling evidence for developing a new classification specific to older adults.

   The prevalence of major depression in nursing homes or long-term care facilities is estimated to be 6%–14.4%, and the prevalence of minor depression to be as high as 30.5%.

   Among women, although the incidence of suicide mortality has long been lower than among men, the age differential in suicide mortality is greater. Older women were 3.22 times more likely to die from suicide than young women (4.9 per 100,000 women ages 15–24 years vs. 15.8 per 100,000 women age 75 years or older) in 2000 (World Health Organization 2000). **(pp. 28–29, 32)**

2.6   A number of genetic and environmental factors may increase the prevalence or age of onset of Alzheimer's disease in seniors. Which of the following statements concerning these factors is **false**?

   A. Persons who are first-degree relatives of someone with Alzheimer's disease are more likely to develop the disease earlier in life.
   B. A family history for dementia was positive for many more patients with Alzheimer's disease compared with individuals who were cognitively intact.
   C. Genetic research in Alzheimer's disease has focused on the APOE*E2 allele.
   D. An association between early-onset Alzheimer's disease and Down syndrome has been reported.
   E. Retrospective studies of the association between head trauma and Alzheimer's disease have found a higher risk of Alzheimer's disease in persons with a history of head trauma.

The correct response is option C.

Genetic research in Alzheimer's disease and dementia has focused on the epsilon 4 allele of the APOE gene (Evans et al. 1997; A.M. Saunders et al. 1993). That is, the ε4 allele (APOE*E4) is a susceptibility gene, in that some (but not all) persons with the allele develop dementia. Some studies have also found a relationship between the APOE*E3 and APOE*E4 alleles and the onset of late-life depression (Krishnan et al. 1996), whereas other studies did not find a link between genotype and change in the number of depressive symptoms (Mauricio et al. 2000).

Heston et al. (1981) studied the relatives of 125 probands who had dementia of the Alzheimer's type (as identified at autopsy). The risk of dementia in first-degree relatives varied with the age of the person at the onset of dementia. Those persons who were first-degree relatives of someone with Alzheimer's disease were more likely to develop the disease earlier in life, suggesting that the inherited form of Alzheimer's disease is associated with an accelerated onset.

Barclay et al. (1986) reported that a family history for dementia was positive in 35.9% of the patients with Alzheimer's disease, compared with 5.6% of the individuals who were cognitively intact.

Investigators have proposed an association between early-onset Alzheimer's disease and Down syndrome, suggesting a common biological or genetic mechanism.

Mortimer et al. (1991) pooled data from 11 retrospective studies and concluded that head trauma increased the risk of Alzheimer's disease (relative risk = 1.82). **(pp. 35–36)**

References

Alexopoulos GS, Meyers BS, Young RC, et al: "Vascular depression" hypothesis. Arch Gen Psychiatry 54:915–922, 1997

American Psychiatric Association: Diagnostic and Statistical Manual of Mental Disorders, 3rd Edition. Washington, DC, American Psychiatric Association, 1980

Barclay LL, Kheyfets S, Zemcov A, et al: Risk factors in Alzheimer's disease, in Alzheimer's Disease and Parkinson's Disease: Strategies for Research and Development. Edited by Fisher A, Hanin I, Lachman C. New York, Plenum, 1986, pp 141–146

Evans DA, Beckett LA, Field T, et al: Apolipoprotein E ε4 and incidence of Alzheimer's disease in a community population of older persons. JAMA 277:822–824, 1997

Federal Interagency Forum on Aging-Related Statistics: Older Americans Update 2006: Key Indicators of Well-Being. Washington, DC, U.S. Government Printing Office, 2006

Heston LL, Mastri AR, Anderson VE, et al: Dementia of the Alzheimer type: clinical genetics, natural history, and associated conditions. Arch Gen Psychiatry 38:1085–1090, 1981

Krishnan KRR, Tupler LA, Ritchie JC, et al: Apolipoprotein E ε4 frequency in geriatric depression. Biol Psychiatry 40:69–71, 1996

Mauricio M, O'Hara R, Yesavage JA, et al: A longitudinal study of apolipoprotein-E genotype and depressive symptoms in community-dwelling older adults. Am J Geriatr Psychiatry 8:196–200, 2000

Mortimer JA, van Duijn CM, Chandra V, et al: Head trauma as a risk factor for Alzheimer's disease: a collaborative re-analysis of case-control studies: EURODEM Risk Factors Research Group. Int J Epidemiol 20 (suppl 2):S28–S35, 1991

National Center for Health Statistics: Health, United States 2006 With Chartbook on Trends in the Health of Americans. Hyattsville, MD, National Center for Health Statistics, 2006

Regier DA, Myers JK, Kramer M, et al: The NIMH Epidemiologic Catchment Area Program: historical context, major objectives and study population characteristics. Arch Gen Psychiatry 41:934–941, 1984

Regier DA, Boyd JH, Burke JD, et al: One-month prevalence of mental disorders in the United States. Arch Gen Psychiatry 45:977–986, 1988

Reynolds CF 3rd, Frank E, Perel JM, et al: Nortriptyline and interpersonal psychotherapy as maintenance therapies for recurrent major depression: a randomized controlled trial in patients older than 59 years. JAMA 281:39–45, 1999

Ritchie K, Artero S, Beluche I, et al: Prevalence of DSM-IV psychiatric disorder in the French elderly population. Br J Psychiatry 184:147–152, 2004

Roses A: Apolipoprotein E affects the rate of Alzheimer disease expression: β-amyloid burden is a secondary consequence dependent on APOE genotype and duration of disease. J Neuropathol Exp Neurol 53:429–437, 1994

Roses A: Genetic testing for Alzheimer disease: practical and ethical issues. Arch Neurol 54:1226–1229, 1997

Saunders AM, Schmader K, Breitner J, et al: Apolipoprotein E ε4 allele distributions in late-onset Alzheimer's disease and in other amyloid-forming diseases. Lancet 342:710–711, 1993

Shoghi-Jadid K, Small G, Agdeppa E, et al: Localization of neurofibrillary tangles and β-amyloid plaques in the brains of living patients with Alzheimer disease. Am J Geriatr Psychiatry 10:24–35, 2002

Steffens DC, Skoog I, Norton M, et al: Prevalence of depression and its treatment in an elderly population: the Cache County study. Arch Gen Psychiatry 57:601–607, 2000

Trollor JN, Anderson TM, Sachdev PS, et al: Prevalence of mental disorders in the elderly: the Australian National Mental Health and Well-Being Survey. Am J Geriatr Psychiatry 15:455–466, 2007

Weissman M, Klerman G: Epidemiology of mental disorders: emerging trends in the United States. Arch Gen Psychiatry 35:705–712, 1978

World Health Organization: Distribution of suicide rates (per 100,000) by gender and age, 2000. Available at http://www.who.int/mental_health/prevention/suicide/suicide_rates_chart/en/index.html. Accessed September 4, 2007.

Chapter 3

Physiological and Clinical Considerations of Geriatric Patient Care

Select the single best response for each question.

3.1 You have a 70-year-old physician patient whom you have treated for a number of years with psychodynamic psychotherapy. She notices that her vision is somewhat impaired around twilight. She asks you about any age-related changes to the eye that may have occurred. Your explanation of age-related changes to the eye that may be impairing her vision at twilight includes all of the following *except*

    A. The pupil becomes more miotic with age.
    B. There is increased curvature of the lens.
    C. The blood vessels of the iris have increased rigidity.
    D. The dilator muscle fibers atrophy.
    E. The lens thickens.

The correct response is option B.

The weakening of the ciliary muscle, combined with decreased curvature of the lens, results in a loss of accommodation; therefore, it becomes difficult for an individual to focus on near objects, and bifocals may be needed.

    The pupil becomes smaller in diameter (more miotic) with age because of atrophy of the dilator muscle fibers and increased rigidity of the blood vessels of the iris. This anatomical alteration in the pupil, combined with the increased thickness of the lens, contributes to the impairment of the visual performance of older persons at twilight. **(p. 46)**

3.2 The heart and blood vessels in the aging patient undergo significant anatomic and physiologic alterations. Which of the following is an example of these changes that occur with aging?

    A. The blood vessels become more distensible.
    B. The intima undergoes significant hypoplasia.
    C. Systolic blood pressure is lower.
    D. There is a decrease in pulse wave velocity.
    E. The cushioning effect of the arterial system is adversely altered.

The correct response is option E.

The ability of arterial vessels to transmit blood is not appreciably affected, but the cushioning effect of the arterial system is adversely altered.

    The heart and blood vessels of aging people undergo significant anatomical alterations. These structural changes lead to changes in function. In addition, age-associated changes in the autonomic nervous system and the response of the cardiovascular system to it have important physiological effects. The ability of the heart to beat faster and pump efficiently and the ease with which blood vessels dilate or constrict are markedly affected. Both cardiac output and cardiac reserves decrease (O'Rourke and Hashimoto 2006; Seals and Esler 2000). With age, human blood vessels stiffen. Anatomically, the intima and media both thicken with age, but according to autopsy studies, this thickening occurs disproportionately in the intima, with intimal hyperplasia observed. The vessels are thicker and less distensible. The physiological results are a greater pulse wave velocity, early reflected pulse waves, and higher systolic blood pressures and aortic pulse pressures in older individuals. Higher pressures can increase the load on the heart and lead to left ventricular enlargement as well as increased left ventricular oxygen requirements, thereby increasing the risk of congestive heart failure. **(pp. 46–47)**

3.3   Your 72-year-old male patient asks you what he could do to improve his respiratory functioning because he has noticed a marked decrease in his respiratory capacity. Although you tell him that respiratory decline cannot be reversed, you recommend which of the following, which has been shown to slow the rate of decline?

    A. Moderate alcohol intake.
    B. Improved sleep hygiene.
    C. Exercise training.
    D. Dietary changes.
    E. Beta-adrenergic blocking agents.

The correct response is option C.

Some studies suggest that exercise training can slow the respiratory decline that occurs with aging. The age-related decrease in maximum oxygen consumption, as well as the decreased responsiveness to low oxygen tension or high carbon dioxide levels, can improve with exercise. Although exercise is helpful, it cannot prevent the ultimate decline in pulmonary function (R.S. Schwartz and Kohrt 2003). **(pp. 47–48)**

3.4   Which of the following changes in endocrine function occurs in elderly patients?

    A. Basal antidiuretic hormone (ADH) levels are normal to increased.
    B. Basal corticotropin levels are decreased.
    C. Aldosterone levels are increased.
    D. Growth hormone levels continue to rise and peak at age 70.
    E. Thyroid function declines significantly leading to an increased risk of hypothyroidism.

The correct response is option A.

Aging causes significant changes in ADH and the body's response to it, which alter the older patient's ability to excrete free water—resulting in hyponatremia—or to prevent volume losses—resulting in dehydration. Basal ADH levels are normal to increased in older adults; because renal free water clearance decreases with age, hyponatremia can more easily occur. However, when volume loss takes place, with subsequent hypotension, less ADH is released in older persons.

Basal corticotropin levels are normal in elderly people. Neither the corticotropin pulse frequency nor its circadian rhythm of secretion is altered. Stimulation of the hypothalamic-pituitary-adrenal axis by exogenous corticotropin produces the expected cortisol response, but the cortisol secretion rate actually declines. Cortisol levels remain the same because of a decrease in the cortisol metabolic clearance rate.

An age-related decrease in plasma renin activity leads to reduced aldosterone secretion; aldosterone levels are thus reduced significantly. The rise in natriuretic hormone secretion in older adults also serves to decrease aldosterone levels; higher levels of natriuretic hormone suppress renin secretion, plasma renin activity, and angiotensin II, further lowering aldosterone secretion. In addition, natriuretic hormone itself can inhibit aldosterone secretion. The ability of corticotropin to stimulate aldosterone secretion is unchanged in the aging adult.

Growth hormone levels peak at puberty and then decrease by 14% per decade. Both a decrease in growth hormone–releasing hormone secretion and an increase in somatostatin are responsible for the decline in growth hormone.

Although there are age-related changes in the thyroid gland, these changes have no corresponding effect on thyroid function. The aging thyroid is more fibrotic and nodular in composition; there have been conflicting reports about whether its size increases, decreases, or remains unchanged. **(pp. 48–50)**

3.5   Aging has no effect upon which of the following pharmacokinetic properties?

     A. Volume of distribution.
     B. Renal clearance rate.
     C. Hepatic drug clearance.
     D. Absorption.
     E. Elimination half-life.

The correct response is option D.

Age has no significant effect on absorption. Although acid secretion, gastrointestinal perfusion, and membrane transport all may decrease and thereby *lower* absorption, gastrointestinal transit time is prolonged and *increases* absorption, and thus no net change occurs.

The volume of distribution is significantly affected by the changes in body mass and total body water that occur with aging. Older patients, with decreased lean body mass and total body water, have a smaller volume of distribution. This is particularly relevant when choosing proper doses for drugs, such as antibiotics or lithium that are primarily distributed in water.

With age, renal mass and renal blood flow are decreased, resulting in a decline in glomerular filtration rate and creatinine clearance. This decrease in clearance can alter the rate at which drugs are excreted, and dosages must be appropriately adjusted.

Hepatic drug clearance is decreased by an age-related decline in hepatic blood flow; oxidative metabolism in the cytochrome P450 system is slower, thereby affecting elimination, but conjugation is not. Underlying hepatic disease and drug interactions also may significantly affect the metabolism of drugs by the liver.

The elimination half-life—the time required for the drug concentration to decrease by half—of certain drugs increases in older adults and may be affected by the relationship between volume of distribution or clearance; this may require adjustment of the drug dosing interval. **(pp. 52–53)**

3.6   Falls in the elderly are unfortunately quite common and are usually multifactorial in origin. By encouraging a patient to improve conditioning and strength through exercise, you are focusing on altering a(n)

     A. Extrinsic factor.
     B. Situational factor.
     C. Psychological factor.
     D. Environmental factor.
     E. Intrinsic factor.

The correct response is option E.

Falls are generally multifactorial and are caused by 1) intrinsic factors, 2) situational factors, 3) extrinsic factors, and 4) medications (Alexander 1999; King and Tinetti 1995). *Intrinsic factors* are disease-specific deficits in an individual patient that might contribute to falling; these factors include neurological problems (central, neuro-muscular, vestibular, visual, and proprioceptive) as well as systemic illness. *Situational factors* relate to the particular activity that is taking place. *Extrinsic factors* relate to the demands and hazards of a particular environment. *Medications* may adversely affect mental status, cognition, balance, circulation, and neuromuscular function and therefore predispose patients to falls.

The prevention of falls focuses on altering both intrinsic and extrinsic factors (Gillespie et al. 2003; King and Tinetti 1995; Rubenstein and Josephson 2006). With regard to intrinsic factors, one can 1) prescribe medication appropriately; 2) optimally treat disease; 3) improve balance and gait through physical therapy; and 4) improve conditioning and strength through exercise.

With regard to extrinsic factors, one can 1) improve the environment by reducing or eliminating hazards; 2) monitor patients more carefully by increasing staff supervision and using motion detection; 3) eliminate restraints and the risk of injury they pose; 4) encourage patients to wear hip protectors; and 5) install protective flooring. Preventing falls ultimately requires multiple steps to produce successful results. **(pp. 54–55)**

3.7 A patient who complains of increased urinary frequency, nocturia, and varying amounts of leakage has which form of established urinary incontinence?

  A. Stress incontinence.
  B. Urge incontinence.
  C. Bladder outlet obstruction.
  D. Detrusor underactivity.
  E. Overflow incontinence.

The correct response is option B.

Urge incontinence has the highest prevalence in older patients. Urge incontinence results from detrusor overactivity, sometimes with simultaneous impaired contractility. Detrusor overactivity is more common with aging but can also occur for other reasons, including neurological dysfunction (e.g., stroke) or irritation of the bladder (secondary to cancer, urolithiasis, or infection); it can also occur in elderly patients without other illnesses. Patients usually complain of a sudden urge to urinate. They also classically have urinary frequency and nocturia. They experience varying amounts of leakage.

Stress incontinence occurs when increased abdominal pressure, triggered by cough or sneezing, results in urinary leakage. It happens commonly in women with weak pelvic muscles, although it also may occur as a consequence of failed anti-incontinence surgery or vaginal mucosal atrophy in women or prostatectomy in men. It is a frequent form of incontinence among elderly women.

Detrusor underactivity and bladder outlet obstruction can both produce overflow incontinence. Detrusor underactivity can be caused by fibrosis of the detrusor muscle, peripheral neuropathy, disc herniation, or spinal stenosis. Detrusor underactivity is an infrequent cause of urinary incontinence in older adults. Urethral strictures, benign prostatic hypertrophy, and prostate cancer can cause bladder outlet obstruction in elderly men; this form of incontinence is the second most prevalent in this population. Bladder outlet obstruction in women occurs much less frequently; the etiology is either the presence of a large cystocele or a history of anti-incontinence surgery. **(pp. 55–56)**

3.8 In men with overflow incontinence, which of the following medications is sometimes prescribed?

  A. Oxybutynin.
  B. Propanolamine.
  C. Alpha-adrenergic blocking agents.
  D. Imipramine.
  E. Tolterodine.

The correct response is option C.

Overflow incontinence in men is most often the result of outlet obstruction due to benign prostatic hypertrophy, which can be treated by both medical and surgical modalities. In clinical trials, α-blockers have been proven most effective for benign prostatic hypertrophy, although finasteride may be used as a second-line treatment.

Urge incontinence is best treated by frequent voluntary voiding and bladder retraining. Patients are placed on a voiding schedule that corresponds to their usual minimal interval of urination. They are taught how to voluntarily inhibit the urge to void. The goal of therapy is to increase gradually the interval between voidings. For patients with cognitive impairment, bladder retraining is not appropriate; instead, timed voiding, scheduled voiding, or prompted voiding is instituted to decrease episodes of incontinence. For those who fail behavioral methods, medications such as oxybutynin, tolterodine, or imipramine may be helpful, but patients should be monitored carefully for anticholinergic side effects. Stress incontinence is also amenable to nonmedical therapy. The mainstay of this approach is to strengthen the pelvic muscles that support the urethra by performing repeated isometric exercises, thereby preventing urinary leakage. Propanolamine also can be a useful adjunct, although this is not an option in patients with hypertension. (p. 56)

References

Alexander NB: Falls and gait disturbances, in Geriatrics Review Syllabus: A Core Curriculum in Geriatric Medicine. Edited by Cobbs E, Duthie EH, Murphy JB. Dubuque, IA, Kendall/Hunt, 1999, pp 145–149

Gillespie LD, Gillespie WJ, Robertson MC, et al: Interventions for preventing falls in elderly people. Cochrane Database Syst Rev Issue 4. Art. No.: CD000340. DOI: 10.1002/14651858.CD000340, 2003

King MB, Tinetti ME: Falls in community-dwelling older persons. J Am Geriatr Soc 43:1146–1154, 1995

O'Rourke MF, Hashimoto J: Mechanical factors in arterial aging: a clinical perspective. J Am Coll Cardiol 50:1–13, 2006

Rubenstein LZ, Josephson KR: Falls and their prevention in elderly people: what does the evidence show? Med Clin North Am 90:807–824, 2006

Seals DR, Esler MD: Human ageing and the sympathoadrenal system. J Physiol 528:407–417, 2000

Schwartz RS, Kohrt WM: Exercise in elderly people: physiological and functional effects, in Principles of Geriatric Medicine and Gerontology, 5th Edition. Edited by Hazzard WR, Blass JP, Halter JB, et al. New York, McGraw-Hill, 2003, pp 931–946

Chapter 4

Neuroanatomy, Neurophysiology, and Neuropathology of Aging

Select the single best response for each question.

4.1   A 67-year-old patient reports a sudden onset of the inability to rotate or tilt his head. You refer him to a neurologist who reports a lesion affecting only the patient's cranial nerve. Which cranial nerve has been affected?

    A. CN VII.
    B. CN IX.
    C. CN X.
    D. CN XI.
    E. CN XII.

The correct response is option D.

The nucleus of the spinal accessory nerve (CN XI) controls the large muscles responsible for rotating and tilting the head.

    The facial motor nucleus (CN VII) controls all the muscles of facial expression.

    The muscles of the larynx and pharynx are controlled by the nucleus ambiguus, with its motor fibers split between the glossopharyngeal (CN IX) and vagus (CN X) nerves.

    The tongue is controlled by the hypoglossal nerve (CN XII). **(p. 65)**

4.2   Which of the following brain stem structures innervates virtually the entire forebrain and is composed of norepinephrine-rich neuronal bodies?

    A. Substantia nigra.
    B. Ventral tegmental area.
    C. Locus coeruleus.
    D. Dorsal raphe nucleus.
    E. Periaqueductal gray.

The correct response is option C.

All three subdivisions of the brain stem contain neuronal cell bodies of the monoamine systems—small groups of cells that together innervate virtually the entire central nervous system (CNS). The monoamines include *norepinephrine* (a catecholamine), which arises from several groups, the largest and most compact of which is the *locus coeruleus*. The locus coeruleus innervates virtually the entire forebrain, giving it the potential to profoundly influence the cerebrum and is considered critical in mood disorders, anxiety, and certain types of drug withdrawal.

A second catecholamine, *dopamine*, arises from the midbrain in a large, compact group known as the *substantia nigra* and from a smaller, diffuse group lying in the anterior tegmental area known as the *ventral tegmental area*. Dopamine deficiencies and excesses figure prominently in certain neurological and psychiatric diseases.

Another monoamine, *serotonin*, is an indoleamine rather than a catecholamine. Some small groups of serotonergic neurons lie throughout the brain stem along the midline anterior to the ventricular system. These collectively are known as the *raphe nuclei*, and individually these groups each innervate certain areas of the CNS from spinal cord to cerebellum to forebrain. The largest and most rostral of the raphe nuclei is called the *dorsal raphe nucleus*, and like the locus coeruleus, it innervates virtually the entire cerebrum, giving the dorsal raphe nucleus the capacity to influence the brain in a global way.

The core of the midbrain is composed of a dense area of neurons surrounding the cerebral aqueduct and is known as the *periaqueductal gray*, an area significantly involved in pain control. **(p. 66)**

4.3   Which of the following brain structures is located at the base of the cerebrum and coordinates endocrine, autonomic, and somatic motor responses to maintain physiological homeostasis?

     A. Hypothalamus.
     B. Thalamus.
     C. Cerebellum.
     D. Pons.
     E. Medulla.

The correct response is option A.

The hypothalamus is a relatively small, heterogeneous structure at the base of the cerebrum. It is roughly divisible into medial and lateral halves, which are extensively interconnected. The hypothalamus plays multiple roles, reflecting its diverse anatomical makeup. Most notably, the hypothalamus serves to coordinate endocrine, autonomic, and somatic motor responses to a broad array of physiological and psychological information to maintain physiological homeostasis. Among the factors regulated by the hypothalamus are body temperature, heart rate, blood pressure, blood osmolarity, metabolism, digestion, and water and food intake. The hypothalamus regulates sexual and reproductive functioning and growth. The hypothalamus also plays roles in the body's responses to stress, including control of adrenal cortical secretion of cortisol, which is part of the body's mechanism for coping with stress. These functions are mediated by a distributed system of interconnected hypothalamic nuclei.

The thalamus is located superior to the hypothalamus, enclosing the upper part of the third ventricle. It is bounded laterally by the white matter of the internal capsule. The thalamus is divided into lateral, medial, and anterior groups by white matter laminae. The thalamus plays a critical role in the functioning of the cerebral cortex. No information enters the cortical mantle without going through the thalamus, with the notable exception of the olfactory system, the most primitive of the sensory systems.

The cerebellum is best known for controlling balance, posture, coordination, and gait. The system is extensive and includes precerebellar nuclei (including the inferior olivary nucleus and several reticular formation nuclei) and their connection to the cerebellum through the inferior cerebellar peduncle.

Although from a gross anatomical perspective, the pons is most notable for the corticocerebellar connections making up the middle cerebellar peduncle, it otherwise is fairly similar to the medulla. The medulla and pons contain the subcortical aspects of the sensory systems for all the cranial nerves (CNs) except CNs I (olfaction) and II (vision). **(pp. 64–65, 67, 68)**

4.4   Deep in the cerebrum are several nuclei constituting the basal ganglia. A multitude of names are given to these structures in various combinations. Which of the following structures comprise the dorsal striatum?

   A. Caudate and globus pallidus.
   B. Putamen and globus pallidus.
   C. Pallidum.
   D. Ventral striatum.
   E. Caudate and putamen.

The correct response is option E.

Deep in the cerebrum are several nuclei constituting the basal ganglia, although a sometimes confusing multitude of names are given to these structures in various combinations. The superior portion of the basal ganglia is known as the *dorsal striatum*, which includes the caudate nucleus and the putamen; these are very similar in structure and essentially split into the two nuclei by fibers of the internal capsule. The striped appearance of the small white matter bundles of the internal capsule and the gray matter bridges still joining the two nuclei in places gave rise to their original, collective name of *striatum* (or rarely *neostriatum*).

   Ventromedial to the putamen are the inner and outer segments of the globus pallidus, making up the third major element of the dorsal striatum. This structure is sometimes just called the *pallidum* (or rarely the *paleostriatum*), so named because the greater content of whitish myelinated axons gives this structure a pale appearance in fresh sections.

   The putamen and globus pallidus are nestled snugly together, giving the appearance of a lens shape with the convex surface oriented laterally and narrowing to somewhat of a point ventromedially, pointing toward the base of the diencephalon. The term *lenticular nucleus* is given to the putamen–globus pallidus combination; this term has usefulness as a gross anatomical term but little usefulness from a functional standpoint.

   The inferior division of the basal ganglia, known as the *ventral striatum*, has a structure that parallels that of the dorsal striatum but differs significantly in connectivity and function. The ventral striatum is usually considered to include the nucleus accumbens and the olfactory tubercle; the nucleus accumbens represents the fused inferior extent of the caudate and putamen. Similarly, the ventral pallidum is the inferior extent of the globus pallidus, so no clear separation exists between dorsal and ventral striatopallidum from a gross anatomical standpoint, although the differences in connectivity clearly justify the nomenclature. **(p. 69)**

4.5   Which of the following structures provides cholinergic innervation to virtually the entire neocortex?

   A. Ventral striatopallidum.
   B. Basal nucleus.
   C. Extended amygdala.
   D. Stria terminalis.
   E. Septal nuclei.

The correct response is option B.

The most diffuse component of the basal forebrain is a system of large cholinergic neurons in a thin disk close to the basal surface of each hemisphere. The most lateral collection of these magnocellular cholinergic neurons is known as the *basal nucleus* (or the basal nucleus of Meynert). The basal nucleus, which receives an extensive and diverse afferent input, provides cholinergic innervation to virtually the entire neocortex, in a manner analogous to the monoamine systems originating in the locus coeruleus and raphe system. The loss of acetylcholine in the cerebral cortex associated with degenerative dementias has been traced to degeneration of this small group of neurons.

The ventral striatum, the inferior division of the basal ganglia, has a structure that parallels that of the dorsal striatum but differs significantly in connectivity and function. The ventral striatum is usually considered to include the nucleus accumbens and the olfactory tubercle; the nucleus accumbens represents the fused inferior extent of the caudate and putamen.

The *extended amygdala* primarily comprises the bed nucleus of the stria terminalis. The stria terminalis is one of two main efferent pathways from the amygdala, and the extended amygdala thus represents a rostral extension of the medial amygdala, with which it shares neurotransmitter properties.

The other magnocellular cholinergic neurons are found in the septal nuclei, the most medial and least diffuse grouping of these neurons. The septal nuclei are part of the limbic system and, with some adjacent neurons, provide cholinergic innervation of the hippocampal formation. **(pp. 69–70)**

4.6   The cerebral cortex can be classified in several different ways. Which category of cortex is characterized by a poorly developed inner granular layer and prominent pyramidal cell layers?

   A. Allocortex.
   B. Association cortex.
   C. Agranular cortex.
   D. Neocortex.
   E. Koniocortex.

The correct response is option C.

A classification scheme was developed by Brodmann based on cytoarchitectonics. Brodmann identified 47 different areas of neocortex, which can be approximately classified into three functional categories. One category is termed *agranular cortex* and is characteristic of motor cortex (Brodmann areas [BAs] 4 and 6). This type of cortex is characterized by a poorly developed inner granular layer and prominent pyramidal cell layers. The large pyramidal cells provide long axons to project long distances to the brain stem or spinal cord.

A second cytoarchitectonic category is termed the *granular cortex* or *koniocortex*, characterized by a prominent inner granular layer and a paucity of large projection neurons. The inner granular layer, so named for the many small neurons concentrated there, is specialized to receive afferent axons and is best developed in sensory cortex.

Another fundamental classification of the cerebral cortex looks at the layering of small and large neurons and neuronal axons in different areas of cortex. Most ($\geq$95%) of the cerebral cortex consists of six layers and is known as *neocortex, isocortex,* or *homotypic cortex.*

Phylogenetically older parts of the cerebral cortex contain fewer layers and are known as *allocortex* or *heterotypic cortex.* The allocortex contains only three layers and includes areas related to olfaction and the hippocampal formation. Notably, whereas the neocortex develops in parallel with the thalamus and receives most of its subcortical afferents from the thalamus, the allocortex receives afferents from other subcortical nuclei.

The large remaining areas of cortex are designated *association cortex,* with variable cytoarchitectonics reflecting both input and output functions.

Brodmann area designations are shown in Figure 4–1 and are related to key regions in Table 4–1. **(pp. 71–72)**

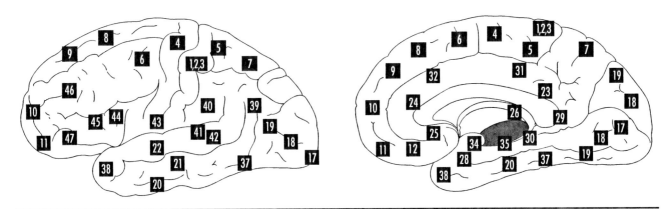

FIGURE 4–1. Illustration of cortical (*left*) and sagittal (*right*) views of the brain, marked with selected Brodmann areas.

TABLE 4–1. Brodmann areas of selected brain regions

Brain region	Brodmann area(s)
Auditory cortex, primary	41, 42
Cingulate cortex	
Dorsal anterior	32
Dorsal posterior	31
Subgenual	25
Ventral anterior	24
Ventral posterior	23
Dorsolateral prefrontal cortex	9, 46
Motor cortex, primary	4
Motor cortex, secondary (premotor, supplementary motor)	6
Orbitofrontal area (orbital gyrus and gyrus rectus)	11
Somatosensory cortex, primary	1, 2, 3
Temporal gyrus	
Inferior	20
Middle	21
Superior	22
Visual cortex, primary	17

4.7   The limbic system is an open system of cortical and subcortical structures with extensive interconnections throughout the central nervous system. Which of the following is one of the cortical limbic structures?

    A. Mamillary nuclei.
    B. Hypothalamus.
    C. Amygdaloid complex.
    D. Hippocampus.
    E. Ventral striatum.

The correct response is option D.

A "limbic system" was originally proposed as the neuroanatomical substrate of emotion. It was conceived as a discrete, closed system of cortical and subcortical structures and addressed the mechanism by which the cerebral cortex influences the hypothalamus and vice versa. As sophisticated tract-tracing techniques have clarified the extensive interconnections between limbic and nonlimbic structures and the existence of distributed systems throughout the CNS, the limbic system is now accepted as an open system thoroughly integrated with structures at all levels of the CNS (Parent 1996).

Cortical regions considered limbic include the parahippocampal gyrus, cingulate gyrus, orbitofrontal cortex, piriform cortex, and hippocampus. The subcortical limbic structures include the amygdaloid complex, ventral striatum, mamillary nuclei, hypothalamus, and several thalamic nuclei. Several limbic structures, including the amygdaloid complex, hippocampal formation, and cingulate gyrus, have extensive interconnections with broad areas of neocortex, including virtually all areas of multimodal sensory association cortex and integrative association cortex. **(p. 75)**

4.8   The EEG of a healthy awake adult is dominated by frequencies in which range?

 A. Delta.
 B. Theta.
 C. Alpha.
 D. Beta.
 E. Chi.

The correct response is option C.

The electroencephalogram of a healthy awake adult is dominated by frequencies in the alpha range. This pattern shows little change with normal aging (Duffy et al. 1984). A small decline in the mean alpha frequency may be seen beginning in the fifth decade, but a significant drop suggests underlying neuropathology.

When comparing healthy subjects across the entire span of the adult years, a small increase in beta frequency activity often correlates with age (Holschneider and Leuchter 1995). Small increases in theta activity are frequently seen in healthy older adults but also may be associated with the subclinical onset of cerebrovascular disease; however, normal aging is generally not associated with significant increases in delta activity (Holschneider and Leuchter 1999).

The spectra of EEG frequencies are conventionally divided into bands defined as delta (<4 Hz), theta (4–8 Hz), alpha (8–13 Hz), and beta (>13 Hz). These frequency bands can be characterized on the basis of *absolute power* (the magnitude of the signal amplitude of a specific frequency band, measured in microvolts squared) and *relative power* (the percent contribution of a specific frequency band to the total power), in addition to measures of ratios of particular frequencies (called *spectral ratios*). **(p. 77)**

4.9   The brain is composed of neurons and supporting cells and structures. Which of the following supporting elements is a complex lipoprotein that serves to protect axonal processes and to facilitate neurotransmission?

 A. Myelin.
 B. Astrocytes.
 C. Oligodendroglia.
 D. Ependyma.
 E. Glia.

The correct response is option A.

Myelin is a complex lipoprotein that serves to protect axonal processes and to facilitate neurotransmission.

The average adult male human brain weighs 1,400 g (Sunderman and Boerner 1949). The organ is composed of neurons and supporting cells and structures. The supporting elements include astrocytes, oligodendroglia, and ependyma, collectively known as *glia*, *blood vessels*, and *myelin*. **(p. 79)**

4.10 Many neurodegenerative processes cause abnormal aggregation of proteins leading to the formation of tangle inclusions in neuronal and glia cells. These proteins are almost entirely made of the protein tubulin and comprise which of the following specialized cell structures?

    A. Lysosomes.
    B. Microtubules.
    C. Lipfusion granules.
    D. Neurofilaments.
    E. Microfilaments.

The correct response is option B.

Microtubules are long, unbranched cylinders composed almost entirely of the protein tubulin (Vogel 1996). Many neurodegenerative processes cause abnormal aggregation or assembly of microtubule-associated proteins.

Neurons are metabolically very active cells and thus require numerous mitochondria. Most of the neuronal mitochondria are contained in the perikaryon. Additionally, numerous proteins are turned over frequently in neuronal cell bodies as a function of their role in synaptic transmission. Some of these proteins are not metabolized entirely, and these nonmetabolized proteins are stored in structures known as *lysosomes*. Histologically, collections of these lysosomes are known as *lipofusion granules*. Increased numbers of lipofusion granules are evidence of normal metabolic wear and tear. As a consequence, they accumulate with age. Microtubules, neurofilaments, and microfilaments are specialized structures that make up the neuronal cytoskeleton. **(p. 80)**

References

Duffy FH, Albert MS, McAnulty G: Age-related differences in brain electrical activity in healthy subjects. Ann Neurol 16:430–438, 1984

Holschneider DP, Leuchter AF: Clinical neurophysiology using electroencephalography in geriatric psychiatry: neurobiologic implications and clinical utility. J Geriatr Psychiatry Neurol 12:150–164, 1999

Parent P: Carpenter's Human Neuroanatomy, 9th Edition. Philadelphia, PA, Williams & Wilkins, 1996

Sunderman FW, Boerner F: Normal Values in Clinical Medicine. Philadelphia, PA, WB Saunders, 1949, pp 641–642

Vogel FS: Neuroanatomy and neuropathology of aging, in The American Psychiatric Press Textbook of Geriatric Psychiatry, 2nd Edition. Edited by Busse EW, Blazer DG. Washington, DC, American Psychiatric Press, 1996, pp 61–70

Chapter 5

Chemical Messengers

Select the single best response for each question.

5.1   Acetylcholine (ACh) acts through a family of muscarinic ACh receptors. Which muscarinic (M) receptor is the most abundant receptor in the neocortex and hippocampus tissue?

    A. M_1.
    B. M_2.
    C. M_3.
    D. M_4.
    E. M_5.

The correct response is option A.

M_1 receptors are the most abundant muscarinic receptors, representing 35%–60% of all muscarinic ACh receptors in neocortex and hippocampus tissue (Levey 1996). M_1 receptors increase norepinephrine release from noradrenergic terminals in the periphery (North et al. 1985; Raiteri et al. 1990), mediate slow excitatory postsynaptic potentials in the ganglions of postganglionic nerves (Xi-Moy et al. 1993), and activate a nitric oxide signal in submandibular glands (Pérez Leirós et al. 1999) that may be relevant to memory and learning ability (Dawson and Dawson 1996).

    ACh acts through the family of muscarinic ACh receptors, of which at least three subtypes (M_1, M_2, and M_3) of the five recognized (M_1–M_5) are involved in the modulation of neurotransmitter release (Caulfield 1993; Caulfield and Birdsall 1998; Raiteri et al. 1990; Starke et al. 1989). M_2 and M_4 receptors are mainly located presynaptically, likely functioning as autoreceptors controlling the release of ACh from the presynaptic neuron terminal. They are found predominantly in the hippocampus and striatum (Levey 1996), where they are able to depress both inhibitory and excitatory neuronal responses. **(p. 96)**

5.2   Which of the following is the major excitatory neurotransmitter in the human brain?

    A. Acetylcholine.
    B. Glutamate.
    C. Gamma-aminobutyric acid.
    D. Dopamine.
    E. Norepinephrine.

The correct response is option B.

Glutamate (or glutamic acid) is the prototypical excitatory neurotransmitter in mammalian brain. Glutamate is also the most ubiquitous transmitter in the mammalian central nervous system (CNS), as nearly every excitatory neuron in the CNS is glutamatergic, and it is estimated that over half of all nerve endings release this amino acid.

    ACh was one of the first biochemicals recognized to be a neurotransmitter. It produces initiation of skeletal muscle contraction and mediates parasympathetic effects and preganglionic autonomic neurotransmission in the peripheral nervous system. ACh is found in cholinergic neurons as well as in the vicinity of cholinergic synapses.

The major inhibitory neurotransmitter in the mammalian CNS is gamma-aminobutyric acid (GABA). GABA is one of the highest-concentration amino acids within the CNS and is synthesized from glutamate by the enzyme glutamic acid decarboxylase.

Dopamine is one of three catecholamine neurotransmitters, the others being norepinephrine and epinephrine. Dopamine is the immediate metabolic precursor of norepinephrine and epinephrine and is formed by the decarboxylation of a previously hydroxylated tyrosine residue.

Norepinephrine, the primary chemical messenger released by postganglionic adrenergic nerves, was originally recognized as a neurotransmitter in the peripheral sympathetic postganglionic fibers and only later found to be a component of the central nervous system. **(pp. 96, 98, 99, 101, 102)**

5.3   The family of serotonin receptors is separated into seven subgroups based on their sequence identities and related functions, with no fewer than 14 individual receptors. Which of the following receptors are decreased by 10% or more per decade in elderly people as compared to young subjects?

   A. 5-HT_{1F}.
   B. 5-HT_{1E}.
   C. 5-HT_{1D}.
   D. 5-HT_{1B}.
   E. 5-HT_{1A}.

The correct response is option E.

Aging-related changes in human serotonin neuronal systems include alterations in levels of specific receptor types and in serotonin transporters. 5-HT_{1A} receptors are decreased by 10% or more per decade in elderly people relative to young subjects (Moller et al. 2007). 5-HT_{2A} receptors are decreased to an even greater degree, with the predominant losses occurring prior to late life (Sheline et al. 2002). **(p. 101)**

5.4   Which of the following neurotransmitters is a substrate for both monoamine oxidase (MAO) and catechol O-methyltransferase (COMT) yielding the metabolic products homovanillic acid and dihydroxyphenylacetic acid?

   A. Serotonin.
   B. Acetylcholine.
   C. Glutamate.
   D. Dopamine.
   E. Histamine.

The correct response is option D.

Dopamine is a substrate for both MAO and COMT, yielding the metabolic products homovanillic acid and dihydroxyphenylacetic acid. Due to its status as a substrate for both MAO and COMT, dopamine itself is ineffective when administered orally. **(p. 101)**

5.5   Which of the following neurotransmitters produces release of stress hormones such as corticotropin-releasing factor and arginine vasopressin?

   A. Serotonin.
   B. Acetylcholine.
   C. Glutamate.
   D. Dopamine.
   E. Histamine.

The correct response is option E.

The role of histamine in allergic responses, as well as in immediate hypersensitivity, is well established, as are the functional uses of histamine receptor antagonists to thwart anaphylaxis and allergy. However, in the CNS, histamine also produces release of stress hormones such as corticotropin-releasing factor and arginine vasopressin. Histamine-containing neurons may participate in the regulation of body temperature, signaling for increased fluid intake, and the secretion of antidiuretic hormone, as well as in the control of blood pressure and the perception of pain. Additionally, histamine may be important for the proper development of the brain, because animal studies indicate that it is one of the first neurotransmitters to appear, and the concentration of histamine is five times higher in prenatal brain than in adult brain. **(p. 103)**

References

Caulfield MP: Muscarinic receptors: characterization, coupling and function. Pharmacol Ther 58:319–379, 1993

Caulfield MP, Birdsall NJ: International Union of Pharmacology, XVII: Classification of muscarinic acetylcholine receptors. Pharmacol Rev 50:279–290, 1998

Dawson TM, Dawson VL: Nitric oxide synthase: role as a transmitter/mediator in the brain and endocrine system. Annu Rev Med 47:219–227, 1996

Levey AI: Muscarinic acetylcholine receptor expression in memory circuits: implications for treatment of Alzheimer disease. Proc Natl Acad Sci U S A 93:13541–13546, 1996

Moller M, Jakobsen S, Gjedde A: Parametric and regional maps of free serotonin $5HT_{1A}$ receptor sites in human brain as function of age in healthy humans. Neuropsychopharmacology 32:1707–1714, 2007

North RA, Slack BE, Surprenant A: Muscarinic M_1 and M_2 receptors mediate depolarization and presynaptic inhibition in guinea-pig enteric nervous system. J Physiol 368:435–452, 1985

Pérez Leirós C, Sterin-Borda L, Hubscher O, et al: Activation of nitric oxide signaling through muscarinic receptors in submandibular glands by primary Sjogren syndrome antibodies. Clin Immunol 90:190–195, 1999

Raiteri M, Marchi M, Paudice P: Presynaptic muscarinic receptors in the central nervous system. Ann N Y Acad Sci 604:113–129, 1990

Sheline YI, Mintun MA, Moerlein SM, et al: Greater loss of $5\text{-}HT_{2A}$ receptors in midlife than in late life. Am J Psychiatry 159:430–435, 2002

Starke K, Gothert M, Kilbinger H: Modulation of neurotransmitter release by presynaptic autoreceptors. Physiol Rev 69:864–989, 1989

Xi-Moy SX, Randall WC, Wurster RD: Nicotinic and muscarinic synaptic transmission in canine intracardiac ganglion cells innervating the sinoatrial node. J Auton Nerv Syst 42:201–213, 1993

C h a p t e r 6

Genetics

Select the single best response for each question.

6.1   Among the fundamental insights to arise from the Human Genome Project is that

A. The number of genes identified encompassed approximately 80% of all DNA.

B. The number of genes was considerably more than expected, currently estimated as 400,000–500,000.

C. The number and function of genes varies widely across mammalian species.

D. The largest proportion of variation within humans and in comparison to other primates is due to structural variations, deletions, and duplications of segments of chromosomes.

E. The silent or noncoding DNA is translated into complex proteins, similar to the genes.

The correct response is option D.

The search for sources of complexity has led to the realization that structural variation, deletions, and duplications of segments of chromosomes make up the largest proportion (at least in terms of numbers of DNA bases) of variation within humans and between humans and other primates (Cheng et al. 2005; Levy et al. 2007).

Among the fundamental insights to arise from the sequencing of the human genome is that the number of genes, currently estimated as 20,000–25,000, was several-fold less than expected, encompassing only about 2% of all DNA. Both the number and function of genes is surprisingly conserved across mammalian species sequenced to date. These findings have caused investigators to look within and across species for other sources of variation, and thus complexity, within the genome. From this has emerged an awareness of the functional roles of the other approximately 98% of the genome, the so-called silent or noncoding DNA (ncDNA), which is never translated into protein. **(p. 119)**

6.2   Diseases caused by genomic rearrangements that result in an altered number of gene copies are often referred to as

A. Single-nucleotide polymorphisms (SNPs).

B. Genomic disorders.

C. Noncoding (nc) DNA errors.

D. Noncoding (nc) RNA errors.

E. Gene transcription disorders.

The correct response is option B.

Diseases caused by genomic rearrangements that result in an altered number of gene copies (copy-number variation [CNV]) are often referred to as *genomic disorders*. Work to map genomic variation in the complete human genome has identified CNV in 1,400 regions that overlap with 14.5% of the genes associated with human disease (Redon et al. 2006).

Until very recently, the majority of known disease-causing mutations have been single DNA nucleotide changes (SNPs) in coding DNA, resulting in altered amino acid sequence of the translated protein. From this has emerged an awareness of the functional roles of the other approximately 98% of the genome, the so-called silent or noncoding DNA (ncDNA), which is never translated into protein. ncDNA sequences are transcribed into noncoding RNA (ncRNA; sequences not functioning as messenger, transfer, or ribosomal RNA) (Carninci et al. 2005). Gene transcription is the process of converting DNA to RNA. **(p. 120)**

6.3   An example of a phenotype that arises from a single-gene disorder is

    A. Early-onset Alzheimer's disease.
    B. Late-onset Alzheimer's disease.
    C. Major depressive disorders.
    D. Bipolar disorders.
    E. Schizophrenia.

The correct response is option A.

Stedman's Medical Dictionary (2005) defines *phenotype* as "The observable characteristics, at the physical, morphological, or biochemical level, of an individual, as determined by the genotype and environment." Phenotypes of interest to geriatric psychiatry that have been the subject of genetic investigation include early- and late-onset Alzheimer's disease, other dementias, major depressive and bipolar disorders, and schizophrenia. Some of these phenotypes, such as early-onset familial Alzheimer's disease, arise from single-gene disorders. However, the majority of these phenotypes, including late-onset Alzheimer's disease, are complex disorders in that they are likely to be influenced by multiple genes, by environmental factors, and by their interaction. **(p. 121)**

6.4   A patient of yours is concerned about her risk of developing late-onset Alzheimer's disease, since her 85-year-old mother has this disorder. What do you tell her is her actual predicted risk of developing Alzheimer's disease?

    A. 31%–40%.
    B. 26%–30%.
    C. 20%–25%.
    D. 15%–19%.
    E. 9%–14%.

The correct response is option D.

Individuals at genetic risk for the development of a disorder in late life may not express the disease symptoms during their lifetime. Late-onset Alzheimer's disease can be used to illustrate this point. It has repeatedly been shown that the first-degree relatives of patients with Alzheimer's disease have a 50% lifetime incidence rate of the disease. However, because of other causes of mortality, it is estimated that only about one-third of this theoretical familial predisposition to Alzheimer's disease is realized in the usual life span (Breitner 1991; Breitner et al. 1988). This means that the actual predicted risk of developing Alzheimer's disease in the first-degree relatives of individuals with Alzheimer's disease is likely between 15% and 19%, compared with 5% in control subjects. Extrapolating from these findings, one could estimate that the risk to children of patients with Alzheimer's disease is one in five or one in six (Liddell et al. 2001). In some cases, the same risk gene, *APOE*E4*, may lead to such competing processes, because the *APOE*E4* genotype predisposes an individual to both cardiovascular disease (Eichner et al. 2002) and Alzheimer's disease (Farrer et al. 1997). **(pp. 121–122)**

6.5   The one gene with a clearly established relationship to late-onset Alzheimer's disease is

    A. Amyloid precursor protein gene (*APP*).
    B. Presenilin-1 (*PS1*).
    C. Apolipoprotein E, ε4 allele (*APOE*E4*).
    D. Presenilin-2 (*PS2*).
    E. Apolipoprotein E, ε2 allele (*APOE*E2*).

The correct response is option C.

The one gene with a clearly established relationship to late-onset Alzheimer's disease is apolipoprotein E, with increased risk of Alzheimer's disease found in individuals carrying the ε4 allele (*APOE*E4*) in both familial and sporadic cases (Brousseau et al. 1994; Mayeux et al. 1993; Rebeck et al. 1993; Saunders et al. 1993; Schmechel et al. 1993). The risk for Alzheimer's disease increases, and the mean age at onset of Alzheimer's disease is earlier, as the number of ε4 alleles an individual carries increases from 0 to 2 (Corder et al. 1993). These findings were confirmed in a meta-analysis of more than 14,000 subjects who were recruited from clinical, community, and brain bank sources, representing multiple ethnic groups (Farrer et al. 1997). Importantly, although the effect of *APOE*E4* on increased risk of Alzheimer's disease was evident in both sexes and in all age and ethnic groups, the magnitude of the risk associated with *APOE*E4* varied by age and ethnicity. Specifically, the risk appeared to be attenuated in older individuals, and in African American and Hispanic individuals (relative to whites). In contrast, the risk conferred by *APOE*E4* was increased in individuals of Japanese ethnicity.

Mutations at three genetic loci associated with early-onset Alzheimer's disease have been identified. The first identified Alzheimer's disease gene was the amyloid precursor protein (*APP*) gene located on chromosome 21 (Goate et al. 1991). Since this first report of a missense mutation (i.e., one amino acid is substituted for another) associated with Alzheimer's disease on this gene, over 20 different missense mutations in *APP* that can cause Alzheimer's disease have been identified (Alzheimer Disease and Frontotemporal Dementia Mutation Database 2008).

A second Alzheimer's disease locus was found on chromosome 14 (St. George-Hyslop et al. 1992; Schellenberg et al. 1992) and is now called presenilin-1 (*PS1*) (Sherrington et al. 1995). More than 160 mutations in the *PS1* locus have now been reported in several hundred families throughout the world (Alzheimer Disease and Frontotemporal Dementia Mutation Database 2008).

A third Alzheimer's disease gene has been localized to chromosome 1 and termed presenilin-2 (*PS2*) (Levy-Lahad et al. 1995a, 1995b). These mutations appear to be rare; only a few families of different ethnicity have been identified with *PS2* mutations. **(pp. 122–124)**

References

Alzheimer Disease and Frontotemporal Dementia Mutation Database. 2008. Available at http://www.molgen.ua.ac.be/ADMutations. Accessed February 13, 2008.

Breitner JC, Murphy EA, Silverman JM, et al: Age-dependent expression of familial risk in Alzheimer's disease. Am J Epidemiol 128:536–548, 1988

Breitner JC: Clinical genetics and genetic counseling in Alzheimer disease. Ann Intern Med 115:601–606, 1991

Brousseau T, Legrain S, Berr C, et al: Confirmation of the epsilon 4 allele of the apolipoprotein E gene as a risk factor for late-onset Alzheimer's disease. Neurology 44:342–344, 1994

Carninci P, Kasukawa T, Katayama S, et al: The transcriptional landscape of the mammalian genome. Science 309:1559–1563, 2005

Cheng Z, Ventura M, She X, et al: A genome-wide comparison of recent chimpanzee and human segmental duplications. Nature 437:88–93, 2005

Corder EH, Saunders AM, Strittmatter WJ, et al: Gene dose of apolipoprotein E type 4 allele and the risk of Alzheimer's disease in late onset families. Science 261:921–923, 1993

Eichner JE, Dunn ST, Perveen G, et al: Apolipoprotein E polymorphism and cardiovascular disease: a HuGE review. Am J Epidemiol 155:487–495, 2002

Farrer LA, Cupples LA, Haines JL, et al: Effects of age, sex, and ethnicity on the association between apolipoprotein E genotype and Alzheimer disease: a meta-analysis. *APOE* and Alzheimer Disease Meta Analysis Consortium. JAMA 278:1349–1356, 1997

Goate A, Chartier-Harlin MC, Mullan M, et al: Segregation of a missense mutation in the amyloid precursor protein gene with familial Alzheimer's disease. Nature 349:704–706, 1991

Levy S, Sutton G, Ng PC, et al: The diploid genome sequence of an individual human. PLoS Biol 5:e254, 2007

Levy-Lahad E, Wasco W, Poorkaj P, et al: Candidate gene for the chromosome 1 familial Alzheimer's disease locus. Science 269:973–977, 1995a

Levy-Lahad E, Wijsman EM, Nemens E, et al: A familial Alzheimer's disease locus on chromosome 1. Science 269:970–973, 1995b

Liddell MB, Lovestone S, Owen MJ: Genetic risk of Alzheimer's disease: advising relatives. Br J Psychiatry 178:7–11, 2001

Mayeux R, Stern Y, Ottman R, et al: The apolipoprotein epsilon 4 allele in patients with Alzheimer's disease. Ann Neurol 34:752–754, 1993

Rebeck GW, Reiter JS, Strickland DK, et al: Apolipoprotein E in sporadic Alzheimer's disease: allelic variation and receptor interactions. Neuron 11:575–580, 1993

Redon R, Ishikawa S, Fitch KR, et al: Global variation in copy number in the human genome. Nature 444:444–454, 2006

Saunders AM, Strittmatter WJ, Schmechel D, et al: Association of apolipoprotein E allele epsilon 4 with late-onset familial and sporadic Alzheimer's disease. Neurology 43:1467–1472, 1993

Schellenberg GD, Bird TD, Wijsman EM, et al: Genetic linkage evidence for a familial Alzheimer's disease locus on chromosome 14. Science 258:668–671, 1992

Schmechel DE, Saunders AM, Strittmatter WJ, et al: Increased amyloid beta-peptide deposition in cerebral cortex as a consequence of apolipoprotein E genotype in late-onset Alzheimer disease. Proc Natl Acad Sci U S A 90:9649–9653, 1993

Sherrington R, Rogaev EI, Liang Y, et al: Cloning of a gene bearing missense mutations in early-onset familial Alzheimer's disease. Nature 375:754–760, 1995

Stedman's Medical Dictionary, 28th Edition. Baltimore, MD, Lippincott Williams & Wilkins, 2005

St George-Hyslop P, Haines J, Rogaev E, et al: Genetic evidence for a novel familial Alzheimer's disease locus on chromosome 14. Nat Genet 2:330–334, 1992

Chapter 7

Psychological Aspects of Normal Aging

Select the single best response for each question.

7.1   Which of the following primary mental abilities declines last with aging but also shows a steeper decline than other abilities from the 70s to the 80s?

   A. Numeric ability.
   B. Inductive reasoning.
   C. Verbal meaning.
   D. Spatial orientation.
   E. Word fluency.

The correct response is option C.

Verbal meaning declines last but also shows steeper decline than the other abilities from the 70s to the 80s (Schaie 2005, p. 116).

   From the extensive longitudinal data on the primary mental abilities used in the Seattle Longitudinal Study (SLS), it can be concluded that the abilities of verbal meaning (recognition vocabulary), spatial orientation, and inductive reasoning reach a peak plateau in midlife from the 40s to the early 60s, whereas number and word fluency peak earlier and show very modest decline beginning in the 50s. The steepness of late-life decline is greatest for number and least for the reasoning ability. More limited data on the multiply-marked latent construct estimates (obtained only in the fifth through seventh study cycles) suggest that peak ages of performance are still shifting and that we now see these peaks occurring in the 50s for inductive reasoning and spatial orientation and in the 60s for verbal ability and verbal memory. By contrast, perceptual speed peaks in the 20s and numeric ability in the late 30s. Even by the late 80s, declines for verbal ability and inductive reasoning are modest, but they are severe in very old age for perceptual speed and numeric ability, with spatial orientation and verbal memory in between (Schaie 2005, p. 127). **(pp. 138–139)**

7.2   At what age will the average older adult's primary mental abilities fall below the middle range of performance for young adults?

   A. 40s.
   B. 50s.
   C. 60s.
   D. 70s.
   E. 80s.

The correct response is option E.

The SLS data suggest that it is during the period of the late 60s and 70s that many people begin to experience noticeable ability declines. Even so, it is not until the 80s are reached that the average older adult will fall below the middle range of performance for young adults. Hence, it turns out that for decisions relating to the retention of individuals in the work force, chronological age is not a useful criterion for groups and is certainly not useful for individuals. This conclusion has of course been the rationale for largely abandoning mandatory retirement in the United States. **(p. 139)**

7.3   Three studies have examined the predictors of the number of days of survival beyond 100 years. Which of the following was a common variable in all three studies that predicted longer survival?

   A. Gender.
   B. Father's age of death.
   C. Residential condition.
   D. Cognitive status.
   E. Nutritional sufficiency.

The correct response is option D.

Poon et al. (2000) examined predictors of number of days of survival beyond 100 years among 105 centenarians from the Georgia Centenarian Study. They found cognition was one of four significant predictors. The others were gender, father's age of death, and nutrition sufficiency. Cognitive status measured by the Short Portable Mental Status Questionnaire was one of five significant predictors of survival among 800 centenarians in the French centenarian study (Robine et al. 2003). The other predictors were residential condition, health status, activities of daily living, and instrumental activities of daily living. Similarly, data from the Tokyo centenarian study (Gondo et al. 2006) showed that Clinical Dementia Rating score had a significant influence on survival. Taken together, these findings indicate cognitive functioning is an important contributor to survival in the general population as well as in the oldest old. **(p. 142)**

7.4   For the clinical psychiatrist, the contributions of neuroimaging research to cognitive changes associated with aging lead to all of the following conclusions *except*

   A. Cognitive change occurs throughout late adulthood.
   B. Some decline in perceptual speed and fluid abilities will be evident only in individuals with early signs of dementias.
   C. Significant changes in brain structure and function may occur in individuals without noticeable cognitive impairment.
   D. Age-related cognitive decline may be minimized to the degree that cardiovascular disease and other comorbidities can be avoided.
   E. The brain is constantly adapting and this adaptation is expressed in measures of older adults' brain function and behavioral measures of cognitive performance.

The correct response is option B.

Cognitive change occurs throughout later adulthood; some decline in perceptual speed and fluid abilities will be evident even in healthy individuals.

Significant changes in brain structure and function may also occur in individuals without noticeable cognitive impairment, although at some point impaired cognitive function will be reflected in the brain measures. Health status is a relevant variable, and to the degree that cardiovascular disease and other comorbidities can be avoided, age-related decline is likely to be minimized. The brain and central nervous system are constantly adaptive, and this adaptation is expressed in measures of older adults' brain function as well as in behavioral measures of cognitive performance. **(pp. 144, 145)**

7.5   Recent research suggests that personality may in fact change over time. Which of the following changes has been reported to occur with aging?

   A. Decrease in neuroticism.
   B. Increase in extraversion.
   C. Decrease in agreeableness.
   D. Increase in openness.
   E. Decrease in conscientiousness.

The correct response is option A.

The unequivocal assertion that personality does not change over time is beginning to be challenged, particularly with the advent of more sophisticated statistical methods that allow for the test of individual growth curves and trajectories. A number of studies have pointed out that neuroticism appears to decline with age (Mroczek and Spiro 2003; Small et al. 2003) and that agreeableness and conscientiousness appear to increase over time (Helson et al. 2002; Small et al. 2003). Terracciano et al. (2005) reported that openness declined across adulthood, neuroticism declined up to age 80, and for extraversion there was first stability and then decline, whereas there was an increase in agreeableness and conscientiousness up to age 70. **(p. 145)**

7.6   A patient asks you whether there are certain personality traits that may predict shorter life spans or premature mortality. Which of the following is such a personality characteristic?

   A. Agreeableness.
   B. Conscientiousness.
   C. Pessimism.
   D. Openness to experiences.
   E. Optimism.

The correct response is option C.

A literature is developing that finds consistent personality mortality associations. Not only does hostility in college predict premature mortality in the University of North Carolina Alumni Heart Study (Siegler 2007), it has also been found that optimists compared with pessimists were more likely to survive 40 years after college entry (Brummett et al. 2006). Friedman and Martin (2007) review conscientiousness as a critical construct in survival and an integrated way to think about personality as a system. The behavioral medicine literature focuses more on negative constructs (hostility, neuroticism, and pessimism), whereas survival studies focus more on the more positive traits. **(p. 147)**

References

Brummett BH, Helms MJ, Dahlstrom WG, et al: Prediction of all-cause mortality by the Minnesota Multiphasic Personality Inventory Optimism-Pessimism Scale Scores: study of a college sample during a 40-year follow-up period. Mayo Clin Proc 81:1541–1544, 2006

Friedman HS, Martin LR: A lifespan approach to personality and longevity: the case of conscientiousness, in Handbook of Health Psychology and Aging. Edited by Aldwin CM, Park CL, Spiro A. New York, Guilford, 2007, pp 167–185

Gondo Y, Hirose N, Arai Y, et al: Functional status of centenarians in Tokyo, Japan: developing better phenotypes of exceptional longevity. J Gerontol A Sci Biol Sci 61:305–310, 2006

Helson R, Jones C, Kwan VS: Personality change over 40 years of adulthood: hierarchical linear modeling analysis of two longitudinal samples. J Pers Soc Psychol 83:752–766, 2002

Mroczek DK, Spiro A 3rd: Modeling intraindividual change in personality traits: findings from the Normative Aging Study. J Gerontol B Sci Psychol Sci 58:P153–P165, 2003

Poon LW, Johnson M, Davey A, et al: Psycho-social predictors of survival among centenarians, in Autonomy Versus Dependence in the Oldest Old. Edited by Martin P, Rott C, Hagberg B, et al. New York, Springer, 2000, pp 77–89

Robine JM, Romieu I, Allard M: [French centenarians and their functional health status] (in French). Presse Med 32:360–364, 2003

Schaie KW: Developmental Influences on Adult Intelligence: The Seattle Longitudinal Study. Oxford, UK, Oxford Press, 2005

Siegler IC: Life course perspective on adult development, in Encyclopedia of Health and Aging. Edited by Markides K. Thousand Oaks, CA, Sage, 2007, pp 324–326

Small BJ, Hertzog C, Hultsch DF, et al: Stability and change in adult personality over 6 years: findings from the Victoria Longitudinal Study. J Gerontol B Sci Psychol Sci 58:P166–P176, 2003

Terracciano A, McCrae RR, Brant LJ: Hierarchical linear modeling analyses of NEO-PI-R scales in the Baltimore Longitudinal Study of Aging. Psychol Aging 20:493–506, 2005

Chapter 8

Social and Economic Factors Related to Psychiatric Disorders in Late Life

Select the single best response for each question.

8.1 A consensual model of the precursors of psychiatric disorders has emerged from the social science and social psychiatry literature. The model is composed of a series of stages. Each of the following is one of these stages *except*

    A. Social integration.
    B. Early events and achievements.
    C. Biological variables.
    D. Provoking agents and copying efforts.
    E. Later events and achievements.

The correct response is option C.

Biological variables are not a factor in the consensual model.

A consensual model of the precursors of psychiatric disorders has emerged in the social science, epidemiological, and social psychiatry literatures. The model remains flexible in terms of specific operationalizations and statistical estimation, but an overarching theoretical orientation has been forged.

The first stage consists of demographic variables that are associated with the risk of psychiatric disorders. Virtually all studies of social factors and psychiatric disorders include demographic factors, especially age, race/ethnicity, and sex. The causal mechanisms that underlie these relationships are unclear, however.

Stage II consists of relatively early experiences that are hypothesized to have persistent effects on an individual's vulnerability to psychiatric disorders. Examples of such experiences include childhood traumas (e.g., the early death or marital disruption of parents) and educational attainment. Stage III consists of later events and experiences, including family relationships and economic achievements. In most studies, stage III indicators are based on the current status of individuals, reinforcing the temporal distinction between stage II and stage III.

Stage IV consists of dimensions of social integration. Social integration occurs at two levels. At the individual level, social integration refers to personal attachments to formal aspects of the social structure (religious affiliation and participation in organizations are two examples). At the aggregate level, social integration refers to the extent to which a collectivity (e.g., a city, a country) is characterized by meaningful ties and a sense of collective identity among residents. **(pp. 158–159)**

8.2 A number of demographic variables have been examined to determine their association with psychiatric disorder in the elderly. Age and gender are two factors that are related to the risk of psychiatric disorders. Which of the following statements concerning age is *true?*

    A. In studies of age differences within the older population, depressive symptoms are lowest among the oldest.

    B. Older adults report levels of depressive symptoms lower than those reported by younger and middle-aged adults.

    C. Some studies have found lower rates of psychiatric symptoms among older adults in comparison to younger adults.

    D. There is a lower lifetime prevalence of depression among older adults.

    E. Older women report lower levels of psychiatric symptoms than men.

The correct response is option D.

Studies of psychiatric disorders (as opposed to symptom levels) demonstrate lower current and lifetime prevalence among older than among younger adults for all nonorganic psychiatric disorders (Robins and Regier 1991). Whether these age differences reflect cohort differences has not been definitively answered. Nonetheless, there is increasing consensus that there are significant cohort effects, as implied by the lower *lifetime* prevalence of depression among older adults. That is, it appears that every new generation exhibits higher rates of depressive disorder than its predecessors (Burke et al. 1991; Kessler et al. 1994; Levenson et al. 1998). The latter two studies report similar patterns for alcohol abuse and dependence.

    Age is related to the risk of psychiatric disorders, but the associations are complex and often inconsistent across studies. Using symptom scales measuring global psychiatric symptoms, a few older studies found higher levels of symptoms among older adults, but most reported the absence of meaningful age differences. Evidence is most plentiful with regard to depressive symptoms. Older adults, especially the very old, usually report levels of depressive symptoms equal to or higher than those reported by younger and middle-aged adults (Blazer et al. 1991; Mirowsky and Ross 1992; Schieman et al. 2002). In studies of age differences within the older population, depressive symptoms are highest among the oldest old (see Cole and Dendukuri 2003 for a meta-analysis).

    Evidence concerning gender differences in psychiatric morbidity is also mixed. Older women report higher levels of psychiatric symptoms, especially depressive symptoms, than do men (Beekman et al. 1999; Hopcroft and Bradley 2007). **(p. 161)**

8.3 Occupation, income, and marriage are important life conditions related to the development of psychiatric disorders. Which of the following statements concerning these life conditions is *false?*

    A. Low income is a risk factor for depressive symptoms.

    B. Retirement increases the risk of developing a psychiatric disorder.

    C. Marital status is weakly associated with psychiatric morbidity.

    D. Remarried women are at significantly higher risk of depression than women married only once.

    E. The unmarried typically report significantly more symptoms of depression than the married.

The correct response is option B.

Retirement is obviously a common transition in later life—a transition that removes individuals from the occupational structure and results in substantial income loss. Nonetheless, there is no evidence that retirement increases the risk of psychiatric disorders (Kim and Moen 2002; Midanik et al. 1995).

    Current and/or recent life conditions also are related to the risk of psychiatric disorder. Income and—to a lesser extent—occupation are related to psychiatric disorder, with low income and low occupational prestige increasing risk during adulthood (Kessler et al. 1994; Robins and Regier 1991). Low income also is a risk factor for both depressive symptoms (Beekman et al. 1999; T. Harris et al. 2003; Kraaij and de Wilde 2001) and the onset of major depressive disorder (Koster et al. 2006) in late life. These relationships are observed using both symptom scales and diagnostic measures. The relationship between marital status and psychiatric disorders remains ambiguous despite considerable research. In general, marital status appears to be weakly associated with psychiatric morbidity, regardless of whether symptom scales or diagnostic measures are used (Robins and Regier 1991). In studies of depression in community-dwelling older adults, the unmarried adults reported significantly more symptoms of depression than did the married adults. Regardless of the cause of the marital dissolution, remarried women were at significantly higher risk for depression than women married only once. **(pp. 162–163)**

8.4   A primary protective factor for the development of psychiatric disorders has been social support. There are several dimensions of social support. One dimension is defined as the specific tangible services provided by families and friends. Which of the following dimensions is so defined?

      A. Social network.
      B. Perceptions of social support.
      C. Informational support.
      D. Level of interaction with family and friends.
      E. Instrumental support.

The correct response is option E.

There is consensus that social support is a multidimensional phenomenon. Most investigators recognize at least three major dimensions: 1) social network—the size and structure of the network of people available to provide support, 2) instrumental support—the specific tangible services provided by families and friends, and 3) perceptions of social support—subjective evaluations of satisfaction with the available support. Some investigators examine a fourth dimension: informational support, defined as the extent to which family and friends provide information that can be used when assessing options and confronting stress. The level of interaction with friends and family and the presence or absence of a confidant also have been examined as indicators of social support. **(p. 164)**

8.5   Compared with current cohorts of older adults, younger adults now are

      A. Less likely to marry.
      B. Less likely to marry for the first time at later ages.
      C. Less likely to divorce.
      D. More likely to have children.
      E. Less likely to have fewer children.

The correct response is option A.

As with education, occupational attainment and income levels are higher among younger than among older cohorts. In light of the documented mental health benefits of higher socioeconomic status, future cohorts of older adults may be at lower risk for psychiatric disorders than are current cohorts. Family formation factors also differ substantially across cohorts. Compared with current cohorts of older adults, younger adults now are less likely to marry, more likely to marry for the first time at later ages, more likely to divorce, less likely to have children, and more likely to have fewer children (Casper and Bianchi 2001). These patterns generate major cohort differences in family size and structure. **(p. 168)**

8.6 In reviewing a number of studies to determine the likelihood of an older adult recovering from depression, you come to several conclusions about factors that may contribute to a poorer outcome. Which of the following factors is associated with a higher likelihood of an older adult's recovering from depression?

    A. Being older.
    B. Being treated in the general medical sector.
    C. Being male.
    D. The recent occurrence of significant life events.
    E. None of the above.

The correct response is option C.

Two groups of depressed older adults have been studied: those who receive treatment in the general medical sector (i.e., from primary care rather than mental health professionals) and those who are untreated. Both groups fare substantially worse in terms of recovery from depression. Cole et al. (2006), for example, reported that 72% of patients treated in the general medical sector do not recover from depression within a year. Beekman et al. (2002) reported that a similar proportion of untreated older adults residing in the community remain depressed 1–3 years later. Both seeking treatment for depression in the general medical sector and obtaining no treatment for depression are common among adults of all ages. Most studies that compared older and younger depressed patients showed no age differences in the likelihood of recovery (Alexopoulos et al. 1996; Andrew et al. 1993; George et al. 1989; Hinrichsen and Hernandez 1993; Mueller et al. 2004). Some studies have found that men are more likely than women to recover from an episode of depression (George et al. 1989; Hughes et al. 1992; Winokur et al. 1993). Four studies reported that the occurrence of life events was associated with a decreased likelihood of recovery (Brugha et al. 1990; Dew et al. 1997; Holahan and Moos 1991; Murphy 1983). **(pp. 169–170)**

8.7 There are a number of reasons why the majority of psychiatric disorders among older adults are treated in the general medical sector. Which of the following is *not* one of these reasons?

    A. Older persons prefer to receive treatment from their primary care physicians.
    B. Medication is greatly preferred over psychotherapy.
    C. Primary care physicians do not refer older patients with psychiatric disorders to mental health professionals.
    D. Older adults are concerned about the stigma of having a psychiatric disorder and needing care.
    E. Older adults have more negative attitudes towards mental health professionals.

The correct response is option B.

There are multiple reasons that the majority of psychiatric disorders among older adults are treated in the general medical sector. First, most older persons prefer to present psychiatric problems to and receive treatment from primary care physicians (Robb et al. 2003). Second, primary care physicians typically do not refer patients with psychiatric disorders to mental health professionals (Gallo et al. 1999). Another barrier to the use of mental health professionals by older adults with mental illness may be resistance by the older adults who need care. Despite decades of public education, the stigma associated with mental illness and receiving care from mental health professionals remains a concern among many Americans (Link et al. 1997). Also, evidence suggests that older adults have more negative attitudes toward mental health professionals than do their younger peers (Robb et al. 2003; Sirey et al. 2001). This barrier is especially disconcerting in light of evidence that in the abstract, older adults report that psychotherapy is greatly preferred over psychotropic medications for emotional problems (Landreville et al. 2001). **(p. 175)**

References

Alexopoulos GS, Meyers BS, Young RC, et al: Recovery in geriatric depression. Arch Gen Psychiatry 53:305–312, 1996

Andrew B, Hawton K, Fagg J, et al: Do psychological factors influence outcome in severely depressed female psychiatric inpatients? Br J Psychiatry 163:747–754, 1993

Beekman AT, Copeland JR, Prince MJ: Review of community prevalence of depression in later life. Br J Psychiatry 174:307–311, 1999

Beekman AT, Gerlings SW, Deeg DJ, et al: The natural history of late life depression: a 6-year prospective study in the community. Arch Gen Psychiatry 59:605–611, 2002

Blazer D, Burchett B, Service C, et al: The association of age and depression among the elderly: an epidemiologic exploration. J Gerontol 46:M210–M215, 1991

Brugha TS, Bebbington PE, Sturt E, et al: The relation between life events and social support networks in a clinically depressed cohort. Soc Psychiatry Psychiatr Epidemiol 25:308–312, 1990

Burke KC, Burke JD Jr, Rae DS, et al: Comparing age at onset of major depression and other psychiatric disorders by birth cohorts in five US community populations. Arch Gen Psychiatry 48:789–795, 1991

Casper LM, Bianchi SM: Continuity and Change in the American Family. Century Oaks, CA, Sage, 2001

Cole MG, Dendukuri N: Risk factors for depression among elderly community subjects: a systematic review and meta-analysis. Am J Psychiatry 160:1147–1156, 2003

Cole MG, McCusker J, Ciampi A, et al: The prognosis of major and minor depression in older medical inpatients. Am J Geriatr Psychiatry 14:966–975, 2006

Dew MA, Reynolds CF 3rd, Houck PR, et al: Temporal profiles of the course of depression during treatment: predictors of pathways toward recovery in the elderly. Arch Gen Psychiatry 54:1016–1024, 1997

Gallo JJ, Ryan SD, Ford DE: Attitudes, knowledge, and behavior of family physicians regarding depression in late life. Arch Fam Med 8:249–256, 1999

George LK, Blazer DG, Hughes DC, et al: Social support and the outcome of major depression. Br J Psychiatry 154:478–485, 1989

Harris T, Cook DG, Victor C, et al: Predictors of depressive symptoms in older people: a survey of two general practice populations. Age Ageing 32:510–518, 2003

Hinrichsen GA, Hernandez NA: Factors associated with recovery from and relapse into major depressive disorder in the elderly. Am J Psychiatry 150:1820–1825, 1993

Holahan CJ, Moos RH: Life stressors, personal and social resources, and depression: a 4-year structural model. J Abnorm Psychol 100:31–38, 1991

Hopcroft RL, Bradley DB: The sex difference in depression across 28 countries. Soc Forces 85:1483–1507, 2007

Hughes DC, Turnbull JE, Blazer DG: Family history of psychiatric disorder and low self-confidence: predictors of depressive symptoms at 12-month follow-up. J Affect Disord 25:197–212, 1992

Kessler D, Lloyd K, Lewis G, et al: Cross-sectional study of symptom attribution and recognition of depression and anxiety in primary care. BMJ 318:436–439, 1999

Kessler RC, McGonagle KA, Zhao S, et al: Lifetime and 12-month prevalence of DSM-III-R psychiatric disorders in the United States: results from the National Comorbidity Survey. Arch Gen Psychiatry 51:8–19, 1994

Kim J, Moen P: Retirement transitions, gender, and psychological well-being: a life-course, ecological model. J Gerontol B Psychol Sci Soc Sci 57:P212–P222, 2002

Koster A, Bosma H, Dempen GLM, et al: Socioeconomic differences in incident depression in older adults: the role of psychological factors, physical health status, and behavioral factors. J Psychosom Res 61:619–627, 2006

Kraaij V, de Wilde EJ: Negative life events and depressive symptoms in the elderly: a life span perspective. Aging Mental Health 5:84–91, 2001

Landreville P, Landry J, Baillargeon L, et al: Older adults' acceptance of psychological and pharmacological treatments for depression. J Gerontol B Psychol Sci Soc Sci 56:P285–P291, 2001

Levenson MR, Aldwin CM, Spiro A 3rd: Age, cohort, and period effects on alcohol consumption and problem drinking: findings from the Normative Aging Study. J Stud Alcohol 59:712–722, 1998

Link BG, Struening E, Rahav M, et al: On stigma and its consequences: Evidence from a longitudinal study of men with dual diagnoses of mental illness and substance abuse. J Health Soc Behav 38:117–190, 1997

Midanik LT, Soghikian K, Ransom LJ, et al: The effect of retirement on mental health and health behaviors: the Kaiser Permanente Retirement Study. J Gerontol B Psychol Sci Soc Sci 50:S59–S61, 1995

Mirowsky J, Ross CE: Age and depression. J Health Soc Behav 33:187–205, 1992

Mueller TI, Kohn R, Leventhal N, et al: The course of depression in elderly patients. Am J Geriatr Psychiatry 12:22–29, 2004

Murphy E: The prognosis of depression in old age. Br J Psychiatry 142:111–119, 1983

Robb C, Haley WE, Becker MA, et al: Attitudes toward mental health care in younger and older adults: similarities and differences. Aging Ment Health 7:142–152, 2003

Robins LN, Regier DA (eds): Psychiatric Disorders in America. New York, Free Press, 1991

Schieman S, Van Gundy K, Taylor J: The relationship between age and depressive symptoms: a test of competing explanatory and suppression influences. J Aging Health 14:260–285, 2002

Sirey JA, Bruce ML, Alexopoulos GS, et al: Perceived stigma as a predictor of treatment discontinuation in young and old outpatients with depression. Am J Psychiatry 158:479–481, 2001

Winokur G, Coryell W, Keller M, et al: A prospective follow-up of patients with bipolar and primary unipolar affective disorder. Arch Gen Psychiatry 50:457–465, 1993

Chapter 9

The Psychiatric Interview of Older Adults

Select the single best response for each question.

9.1 In gathering information from elderly patients concerning their present illness, you should assess their function and change in function. Two important parameters for this type of assessment are not normally included in the assessment of physical and psychiatric illness in younger adults. One of these parameters is social functioning. What is the other?

    A. Alcohol use.
    B. Current medications.
    C. Employment.
    D. Activities of daily living.
    E. Educational achievement.

The correct response is option D.

The two parameters that are most important (and not included in usual assessments of physical and psychiatric illness) are social functioning and activities of daily living (ADLs). Questions should be asked about the social interaction of the older adult, such as the frequency of his or her visits outside the home, telephone calls, and visits from family and friends. Many scales have been developed to assess ADLs; however, in the interview, the clinician can simply ask about the patient's ability to get around (e.g., walk inside and outside the house), to perform certain physical activities independently (e.g., bathe, dress, shave, brush teeth, and select clothes), and to do instrumental activities (e.g., cook, maintain a bank account, shop, and drive). It is also important to assess how often the elder actually engages in these activities; for example, the ability to walk outside does not always translate to outdoor exercise. **(pp. 188–189)**

9.2 A primary goal of the clinician as an advocate for the psychiatrically ill older adult is to facilitate family support. Areas that are important to evaluate include all of the following *except*

    A. Whether a family member has a similar psychiatric disorder.
    B. Tolerance by the family of specific behavior related to the psychiatric disorder.
    C. The tangible services that may be provided by the family.
    D. Availability of family members.
    E. Perceptions of family support by the older patient.

The correct response is option A.

At least four parameters of support are important for the clinician to evaluate as the treatment plan evolves: 1) the availability of family members to the older person over time; 2) the tangible services provided by the family to the older person; 3) the perception of family support by the older patient (and therefore the willingness of the patient to cooperate and accept support); and 4) tolerance by the family of specific behaviors that derive from the psychiatric disorder. **(p. 190)**

9.3   Testing the memory of an older patient is an important component of the mental status examination. Asking the older person to repeat a word, phrase, or series of numbers assesses which component of memory?

    A. Registration.
    B. Retention.
    C. Immediate recall.
    D. Orientation.
    E. Distant memory.

The correct response is option C.

Testing of memory is based on three essential processes: 1) registration (the ability to record an experience in the central nervous system), 2) retention (the persistence and permanence of a registered experience), and 3) recall (the ability to summon consciously the registered experience and report it) (Linn 1980).

Disturbances of recall can be tested directly in a number of ways. The most common are *tests of orientation* to time, place, person, and situation. Most persons continually orient themselves through radio, television, and reading material, as well as through conversations with others. Some elderly persons may be isolated through sensory impairment or lack of social contact; poor orientation in these patients may represent deficits in the physical and social environment rather than brain dysfunction. *Immediate recall* can be tested by asking the older person to repeat a word, phrase, or series of numbers, but it can also be tested in conjunction with cognitive skills by requesting that a word be spelled backward or that elements of a story be recalled.

Registration, apart from recall, is difficult to evaluate directly. Occasionally, events or information that the older adult denies remembering will appear spontaneously during other parts of the interview. Registration usually is not impaired, except in patients with one of the more severely dementing illnesses.

Retention, on the other hand, can be blocked by both psychic distress and brain dysfunction. Lack of retention is especially relevant to the unimportant data often asked for on a mental status examination. For example, requesting the older adult to remember three objects for 5 minutes will frequently reveal a deficit if the older adult has little motivation to attempt the task. **(p. 193)**

9.4   A number of rating scales have been used to screen for depression in seniors. Which of the following is an interviewer-rated scale that does **not** include many of the somatic symptoms that tend to be more common in older adults?

    A. Center for Epidemiologic Studies Depression Scale (CES-D).
    B. Montgomery-Åsberg Rating Scale for Depression.
    C. Beck Depression Inventory (BDI).
    D. Geriatric Depression Scale (GDS).
    E. Hamilton Rating Scale for Depression (Ham-D).

The correct response is option B.

A scale that has received considerable attention clinically, having been standardized in clinical but not community populations, is the Montgomery-Åsberg Rating Scale for Depression (Montgomery and Åsberg 1979). This scale follows the pattern of the Hamilton scale and concentrates on 10 symptoms of depression; the clinician rates each symptom on a scale of 0–6 (for a range of scores between 0 and 60). The symptoms include apparent sadness, reported sadness, inattention, reduced sleep, reduced appetite, concentration difficulties, lassitude, inability to feel, pessimistic thoughts, and suicidal thoughts. The instrument does not include many somatic symptoms that tend to be more common in older adults, and therefore it may be of greater value in tracking the symptoms of depressive illness that would be expected to change with therapy.

The most widely used of the current instruments in community studies is the Center for Epidemiologic Studies Depression Scale (CES-D) (Radloff 1977). The scale consists of 20 behaviors and feelings, and the patient indicates how frequently each was experienced over the past week (from no days to most days).

A scale that has been widely used in clinical studies, although less studied in community populations, is the Beck Depression Inventory (BDI) (Beck et al. 1961). The reliability of the BDI has been shown to be good in both depressed and nondepressed samples of older people (Gallagher et al. 1982). The instrument consists of 21 symptoms and attitudes, rated on a scale of 0–3 in terms of intensity.

The Geriatric Depression Scale (GDS) was developed because the scales discussed above present problems for older persons who have difficulty in selecting one of four forced-response items (Yesavage et al. 1983). The GDS is a 30-item scale that permits patients to rate items as either present or absent; it includes questions about symptoms such as cognitive complaints, self-image, and losses. Items selected were thought to have relevance to late-life depression.

Of the scales used by interviewers to rate patients, the Hamilton Rating Scale for Depression (Ham-D) (Hamilton 1960) is by far the most commonly used. The advantage of having ratings based on clinical judgment has made the Ham-D a popular instrument for rating outcome in clinical trials. (pp. 194–195)

9.5   Which of the following general assessment scales produces functional impairment ratings in five areas: mental health, physical health, social functioning, economic functioning, and activities of daily living?

   A. Global Assessment of Functioning Scale.
   B. Geriatric Mental State Schedule.
   C. Psychiatric Status Schedule.
   D. Comprehensive Assessment and Referral Evaluation.
   E. Older Americans Resources and Services (OARS) Multidimensional Functional Assessment Questionnaire.

The correct response is option E.

The OARS Multidimensional Functional Assessment Questionnaire (Duke University Center for the Study of Aging and Human Development 1978), administered by a lay interviewer, produces functional impairment ratings in five dimensions: mental health, physical health, social functioning, economic functioning, and activities of daily living.

One of the more frequently used scales of psychiatric status is the Global Assessment of Functioning Scale (American Psychiatric Association 2000). Using this scale, the rater makes a single rating, from 0 to 100, that best describes—on the basis of his or her clinical judgment—the lowest level of the subject's functioning in the week before the rating. The scale has not been standardized for older adults, but its common use in psychiatric studies suggests the need for standardization.

The Geriatric Mental State Schedule (Copeland et al. 1976), an adaptation of the Present State Exam (Wing et al. 1974) and the Psychiatric Status Schedule (Spitzer et al. 1968), is a semistructured interviewing guide that allows the rater to inventory symptoms associated with psychiatric disorders. More than 500 ratings are made on the basis of information obtained by a highly trained interviewer, who elicits reports of symptoms from the month preceding the evaluation.

The Comprehensive Assessment and Referral Evaluation (Gurland et al. 1977) is a hybridized assessment procedure developed for older adults. Dimensional scores are obtained in these areas: Memory–Disorientation, Depression–Anxiety, Immobility–Incapacity, Isolation, Physical–Perceptual Difficulty, and Poor Housing–Income. (pp. 195–196)

9.6   In interviewing an older patient, psychiatrists may apply a variety of techniques to improve communication. In general, which of the following techniques should ***not*** be used in older adults?

   A. Speak clearly and slowly, since many seniors have hearing difficulties.
   B. Take a position near the older person.
   C. Address the person by surname to demonstrate respect.
   D. Avoid silent pauses, since elders get uncomfortable with silence.
   E. Allow the senior enough time to respond to questions.

The correct response is option D.

Certain techniques have generally proved to be valuable in communicating with the elderly patient. These techniques should not be implemented indiscriminately, however, for the variation among the population of older adults is significant. First, the older person should be approached with respect. The clinician should knock before entering a patient's room and should greet the patient by surname (e.g., Mr. Jones, Mrs. Smith) rather than by a given name, unless the clinician also wishes to be addressed by a given name. After taking a position near the older person—near enough to reach out and touch the patient—the clinician should speak clearly and slowly and use simple sentences in case the person's hearing is impaired. Because of hearing problems, older patients may understand conversation better over the telephone than in person. By placing the receiver against the mastoid bone, the patient with otosclerosis can take advantage of preserved bone conduction. The interview should be paced so that the older person has enough time to respond to questions. Most elders are not uncomfortable with silence, because it gives them an opportunity to formulate their answers to questions and elaborate certain points they wish to emphasize. Nonverbal communication is frequently a key to effective communication with elderly persons, because they may be reticent about revealing affect verbally. The patient's facial expressions, gestures, postures, and long silences may provide clues to the clinician about issues that are unspoken. One key to successful communication with an older adult is a willingness to continue working as a professional with that person. Older adults—possibly unlike some of their children and grandchildren—place a great deal of stress on loyalty and continuity. Most elderly patients do not require large amounts of time from clinicians, and with those who are more demanding, such needs can usually be controlled through structure in the interview. **(p. 197)**

References

American Psychiatric Association: Diagnostic and Statistical Manual of Mental Disorders, 4th Edition, Text Revision. Washington, DC, American Psychiatric Association, 2000

Beck AT, Ward CH, Mendelson M, et al: An inventory for measuring depression. Arch Gen Psychiatry 4:561–571, 1961

Copeland JR, Kelleher MJ, Kellett JM, et al: A semi-structured clinical interview for the assessment and diagnosis of mental state in the elderly: the Geriatric Mental State Schedule. I. Development and reliability. Psychol Med 6:439–449, 1976

Duke University Center for the Study of Aging and Human Development: Multidimensional Functional Assessment: The OARS Methodology—A Manual, 2nd Edition. Durham, NC, Duke University Center for the Study of Aging and Human Development, 1978

Gallagher D, Nies G, Thompson LW: Reliability of the Beck Depression Inventory with older adults. J Consult Clin Psychol 50:152–153, 1982

Gurland B, Kuriansky J, Sharpe L, et al: The Comprehensive Assessment and Referral Evaluation (CARE)—rationale, development and reliability. Int J Aging Hum Dev 8:9–42, 1977

Hamilton M: A rating scale for depression. J Neurol Neurosurg Psychiatry 23:56–62, 1960

Linn L: Clinical manifestations of psychiatric disorders, in Comprehensive Textbook of Psychiatry, 3rd Edition, Vol 1. Edited by Kaplan HI, Freedman AM, Sadock BJ. Baltimore, MD, Williams and Wilkins, 1980, pp 990–1034

Montgomery SA, Åsberg M: A new depression scale designed to be sensitive to change. Br J Psychiatry 134:382–389, 1979

Radloff LS: The CES-D Scale: a self-report depression scale for research in the general population. Applied Psychological Measurement 1:385–401, 1977

Spitzer RL, Endicott J, Cohen GM: Psychiatric Status Schedule, 2nd Edition. New York, New York State Department of Mental Hygiene, Evaluation Unit, Biometrics Research, 1968

Wing JK, Cooper JE, Sartorius N: The Measurement and Classification of Psychiatric Symptoms. London, Cambridge University Press, 1974

Yesavage JA, Brink TL, Rose TL, et al: Development and validation of a geriatric depression screening scale: a preliminary report. J Psychiatr Res 17:37–49, 1983

C h a p t e r   1 0

Use of the Laboratory in the Diagnostic Workup of Older Adults

Select the single best response for each question.

10.1 You are treating an 83-year-old patient for depression and she develops fatigue, nausea, dizziness, gait disturbances, forgetfulness, confusion, lethargy, and muscle cramps. You obtain a general chemistry panel, and her serum sodium concentration is 120 mEq/L. What psychotropic medication has been reported to produce this condition in the elderly?

  A. Bupropion.
  B. Selective serotonin reuptake inhibitors.
  C. Depakote.
  D. Venlafaxine.
  E. Tricyclic antidepressants.

The correct response is option B.

Hyponatremia—commonly defined as a serum sodium concentration less than 135 mEq/L—has been reported with selective serotonin reuptake inhibitors (SSRIs), particularly in the elderly (Jacob and Spinler 2006). The signs and symptoms of hyponatremia result from neurological dysfunction secondary to cerebral edema. Acute hyponatremia can start with nausea and malaise when the plasma sodium concentration falls below 125–130 mEq/L and can progress rapidly to coma and respiratory arrest if the plasma sodium concentration falls below 115–120 mEq/L. In chronic hyponatremia, the brain cells adapt to the edema and symptoms are much less severe. Patients may be asymptomatic despite a plasma sodium concentration that is persistently as low as 115–120 mEq/L. When symptoms do occur in patients with low sodium concentrations, they are relatively nonspecific (e.g., fatigue, nausea, dizziness, gait disturbances, forgetfulness, confusion, lethargy, muscle cramps). The clinician should be vigilant to this risk in older adults started on SSRIs. **(p. 202)**

10.2 You are asked to evaluate a 79-year-old man who was hospitalized on the general medical service for evaluation of mental status changes associated with malnutrition. You recommend to the medical team that they order a serum homocysteine level. The resident asks why the order is necessary. All of the following answers are true *except*

  A. Hyperhomocysteinemia is prevalent in the elderly.
  B. High levels of homocysteine can be attributed to an inadequate supply of B_{12} and folate.
  C. Hyperhomocysteinemia is associated with cognitive dysfunction.
  D. High levels of homocysteine have been associated with an increased risk for occlusive vascular disease, thrombosis, and stroke.
  E. Vitamin supplementation to reduce plasma homocysteine has been shown in numerous studies to improve cognition.

The correct response is option E.

Results on whether vitamin supplementation to reduce plasma homocysteine levels also leads to improved cognition are mixed, with some studies showing benefit (Durga et al. 2007; Nilsson et al. 2001) and others showing no benefit despite lowered homocysteine levels (McMahon et al. 2006).

Serum homocysteine levels may serve as a functional indicator of B_{12} and folate status (Selhub et al. 2000), because both vitamins are needed to convert homocysteine to methionine in one-carbon metabolism in brain tissue. Hyperhomocysteinemia is prevalent in elderly persons, and high serum levels of homocysteine can be attributed to an inadequate supply of B_{12} and folate, even in the presence of low normal serum levels (Selhub et al. 2000). High levels of homocysteine have also been associated with increased risk of occlusive vascular disease, thrombosis, and stroke (Boushey et al. 1995). Hyperhomocysteinemia is further associated with cognitive dysfunction (Leblhuber et al. 2000; Selhub et al. 2000), although not all authors have found this association (Ravaglia et al. 2000). In a longitudinal study of 965 older individuals, a lower incidence of Alzheimer's disease was noted among those subjects in the highest quartile of total folate intake, after adjustments for age, sex, education, ethnicity, and other comorbidities. Neither vitamin B_6 nor vitamin B_{12} intake was associated with risk of Alzheimer's disease (Luchsinger et al. 2007). **(p. 204)**

10.3   In a community psychiatry clinic, you see for the first time a 78-year-old patient who has been treated for a number of years with thioridazine. You immediately decide to order an electrocardiogram (ECG). What ECG changes are you particularly concerned about?

   A. Atrioventricular block.
   B. Sinoatrial block.
   C. QTc prolongation.
   D. PR internal prolongation.
   E. Prolonged QRS complex.

The correct response is option C.

Antipsychotics can result in electrocardiographic changes; about 25% of individuals receiving antipsychotics exhibit electrocardiographic abnormalities (Thomas 1994). Although many of these changes have historically been considered benign, there is increased concern that prolongation of the QT interval may contribute to potentially fatal ventricular arrhythmias, particularly torsades de pointes. This phenomenon may be seen with almost any antipsychotic agent but is most likely to be associated with thioridazine and haloperidol among typical antipsychotics and with ziprasidone among atypical antipsychotics (Glassman and Bigger 2001).

Although the most common cardiovascular complication of tricyclic antidepressants (TCAs) is orthostatic hypotension (Glassman and Bigger 1981), TCAs have the same pharmacological properties as type IA antiarrhythmics, such as quinidine and procainamide. TCAs slow conduction at the bundle of His; individuals with preexisting bundle branch block who take TCAs are at increased risk for atrioventricular block. Even therapeutic levels are associated with prolonged PR intervals and QRS complexes; these results may be more pronounced in elderly individuals because the incidence and severity of adverse drug reactions increase with age (Pollock 1999). If TCAs are used, baseline and frequent follow-up ECGs should be obtained.

Lithium appears to most affect the sinus node, and even at therapeutic levels it may result in sick sinus syndrome or sinoatrial block, either of which may occur early or later in treatment. **(pp. 205–206)**

10.4 When used to examine brain structures, computed tomography (CT) is an effective radiographic technique. However, it does have limitations. Which of the following is a major limitation?

    A. It cannot demonstrate bone abnormalities such as skull fractures.
    B. It is not effective in detecting subdural hematomas.
    C. It is ineffective in showing the mass effect from various lesions.
    D. It does not visualize posterior fossa structures well because of surrounding bone.
    E. It cannot demonstrate ventricular enlargement.

The correct response is option D.

When used to examine brain structure, computed tomography can allow for the ready identification of many structures, although it does have limitations. By measuring differences in density, it can distinguish among cerebrospinal fluid (CSF), blood, bone, gray matter, and white matter. CT is particularly useful for demonstrating bone abnormalities (such as skull fractures), areas of hemorrhage (such as a subdural hematoma), and the mass effect from various lesions. It can also display atrophy or ventricular enlargement. However, CT is not very useful for visualizing posterior fossa or brain stem structures because of surrounding bone. **(p. 207)**

10.5 When compared with CT imaging, magnetic resonance imaging (MRI) has advantages and disadvantages. All of the following are disadvantages of MRI, as compared to CT, *except*

    A. Radiation is used.
    B. The procedure takes longer.
    C. It is usually more costly.
    D. The device must be housed in an area devoid of iron.
    E. Patients cannot carry or wear certain metals or have them embedded in their bodies.

The correct response is option A.

MRI has advantages and disadvantages when compared with CT imaging. MRI produces higher-resolution images and can obtain good detail in regions (such as the posterior fossa) that are poorly visualized on CT. Additionally, no radiation is involved. Unfortunately, the procedure is more grueling than CT because the patient must remain motionless for a longer period of time in a smaller, enclosed space. This may be difficult for claustrophobic individuals. Additionally, the magnetic device must be housed in an area devoid of iron, and staff and patients must not carry or wear certain metals or have them embedded in their bodies. Moreover, MRI tends to be more costly than CT imaging in most institutions. **(p. 207)**

References

Boushey CJ, Beresford SA, Omenn GS, et al: A quantitative assessment of plasma homocysteine as a risk factor for vascular disease: probable benefits of increasing folic acid intakes. JAMA 274:1049–1057, 1995

Durga J, van Boxtel MP, Schouten EG, et al: Effect of 3-year folic acid supplementation on cognitive function in older adults in the FACIT trial: a randomised, double blind, controlled trial. Lancet 369:208–216, 2007

Glassman AH, Bigger JT Jr: Cardiovascular effects of therapeutic doses of tricyclic antidepressants: a review. Arch Gen Psychiatry 38:815–820, 1981

Glassman AH, Bigger JT: Antipsychotic drugs: prolonged QTc interval, torsades de pointes, and sudden death. Am J Psychiatry 158:1774–1782, 2001

Jacob S, Spinler SA: Hyponatremia associated with selective serotonin-reuptake inhibitors in older adults. Ann Pharmacother 40:1618–1622, 2006

Leblhuber F, Walli J, Artner-Dworzak E, et al: Hyperhomocysteinemia in dementia. J Neural Transm 107:1469–1474, 2000

Luchsinger JA, Tang MX, Miller J, et al: Relation of higher folate intake to lower risk of Alzheimer disease in the elderly. Arch Neurol 64:86–92, 2007

McMahon JA, Green TJ, Skeaff CM, et al: A controlled trial of homocysteine lowering and cognitive performance. N Engl J Med 354:2764–2772, 2006

Nilsson K, Gustafson L, Hultberg B: Improvement of cognitive functions after cobalamin/folate supplementation in elderly patients with dementia and elevated plasma homocysteine. Int J Geriatr Psychiatry 16:609–614, 2001

Pollock BG: Adverse reactions of antidepressants in elderly patients. J Clin Psychiatry 60:4–8, 1999

Ravaglia G, Forti P, Maioli F, et al: Elevated plasma homocysteine levels in centenarians are not associated with cognitive impairment. Mech Ageing Dev 121:251–261, 2000

Selhub J, Bagley LC, Miller J, et al: B vitamins, homocysteine, and neurocognitive function in the elderly. Am J Clin Nutr 71(suppl):614S–620S, 2000

Thomas SH: Drugs, QT interval abnormalities, and ventricular arrhythmias. Adverse Drug React Toxicol Rev 13:77–102, 1994

Chapter 11

Neuropsychological Assessment of Dementia

Select the single best response for each question.

11.1 Age-related cognitive changes are manifested in the decline in a number of tasks or abilities. Which of the following cognitive processes are less susceptible to age?

    A. Motor responses.
    B. Crystallized skills.
    C. Reaction times.
    D. Fluid abilities.
    E. Retrieval functions.

The correct response is option B.

A number of explanations for age-related cognitive change have been suggested, none of which are mutually exclusive. All basically support a premise of a broad explanatory mechanism for age-related cognitive change rather than unique and specific changes in restricted cognitive domains. Speed of central processing has been one popular unifying notion, given that the majority of tasks affected in aging involve motor responses or reaction times (Salthouse 2005). Recent empirical studies support slowed central processing as a leading explanation for cognitive change with aging (Finkel et al. 2007). Another explanation posits that the profile of cognitive change in normal aging is the result of a loss in "fluid" abilities, skills that require novel problem solving and flexible thought (Botwinick 1977; Horn 1982). Well-rehearsed verbal abilities ("crystallized" skills), by contrast, are less susceptible to age-associated change. More contemporary refinements of this hypothesis conceptualize normal aging as a selective vulnerability in frontal, dysexecutive processes (Daigneault and Braun 1993; Mittenberg et al. 1989; Van Gorp and Mahler 1990). This notion is consistent with the behavioral difficulties observed, suggesting subtle impairments in integrative and retrieval functions, and is also supported by neuroimaging (Coffey et al. 1992; Gur et al. 1987; Langley and Madden 2000; Tisserand 2003) and histopathological findings (Haug et al. 1983) within the frontal-subcortical brain connections. **(p. 216)**

11.2 In the early stages of Alzheimer's disease, the medial temporal lobe is most affected, leading to impairment of which of the following cognitive processes?

    A. Recent memory.
    B. Expressive language.
    C. Visuospatial function.
    D. Higher executive control.
    E. Semantic knowledge.

The correct response is option A.

The presentation of Alzheimer's disease dementia is dominated by a pronounced impairment in recent memory processing, and this remains the most affected area of mentation in the majority of cases. This difficulty is now understood to arise from the selective involvement of the medial temporal lobe early in the illness (Braak and Braak 1991; Hyman et al. 1984), giving rise to impaired consolidation of newly learned information into more permanent memory stores located across interconnected neocortical structures.

As the disease progresses, other areas of cognition become progressively more involved, reflecting the specific spread of neuropathological involvement to the lateral temporal areas, parietal cortex, and frontal neocortical areas (Small et al. 2000; Storandt et al. 2006; Welsh et al. 1992). Prototypical changes occur in expressive language, visuospatial function, higher executive control, and semantic knowledge (Locascio et al. 1995; Mickes et al. 2007; Storandt et al. 2006). At these latter stages of the illness, anomia with impaired semantic fluency (e.g., generation of names of animals) is generally seen on examination. Word search and circumlocution tendencies are common in conversational speech, whereas speech comprehension itself is better preserved, as are all other fundamental elements of communication (Bayles et al. 1989). Visuospatial problems become more prominent in later stages of illness, resulting in dressing apraxia, difficulty in recognizing objects or people, and problems in performing familiar motor acts (Benke 1993). **(pp. 216–218)**

11.3 Which of the following dementias is characterized by early fluctuations in cognition and attention, recurrent and persistent visual hallucinations, and extrapyramidal motor symptoms?

    A. Alzheimer's disease.
    B. Frontotemporal lobar dementia (FTLD).
    C. Dementia with Lewy bodies (DLB).
    D. Parkinson's disease dementia (PDD).
    E. Vascular dementia.

The correct response is option C.

DLB, a progressive neurological condition, is heralded by cognitive, behavioral, and functional impairments, as opposed to extrapyramidal motor symptoms, and is associated with a disorder of α-synuclein metabolism. The recent recognition that DLB and PDD share a common biology has led to their being grouped together and referred collectively as "Lewy body dementia" (LBD). In LBD, the prevailing features are parkinsonism, akinetic rigidity, and generalized slowing in motor movement/initiation and thought processes, bradykinesia and bradyphrenia, respectively. DLB, in contrast, is characterized by early fluctuations in cognition and attention, recurrent and persistent visual hallucinations, and extrapyramidal motor symptoms. In PDD, symptoms of dementia emerge in the context of a previously established diagnosis of Parkinson's disease, whereas in LBD, the symptoms of cognitive and functional impairments either predate or follow the onset of parkinsonian symptoms within a 1-year time interval.

FTLD refers to a heterogeneous group of neurodegenerative conditions that are now recognized as a major non–Alzheimer's disease dementia. Typically the onset of disease is in the presenium, distinguishing it from Alzheimer's disease where the typical age of onset occurs to appear later, after age 65. The exact prevalence of FTLD remains inconclusive in late old age, but recent studies suggest that it accounts for approximately 10%–20% of the early-onset dementias (Ratnavalli et al. 2002; Snowden et al. 2002).

Patients with Parkinson's disease commonly have cognitive complaints and many go on to develop dementia. Although the cumulative prevalence estimates of PDD remain unclear, recent estimates suggest that 10%–30% of newly diagnosed Parkinson's disease patients develop dementia within 3 years (Reid et al. 1996; Williams-Gray et al. 2007).

The neuropsychological profile of vascular dementia differs in many respects from that of Alzheimer's disease, the largest difference being the absence of the profound memory impairment that is a hallmark of the latter disorder (Tierney et al. 2001). The presentation will vary according to the type and extent of the vascular disorder, be it multiple infarctions, a single strategic stroke, microvascular disease, cerebral hypoperfusion, hemorrhage, or combinations of these etiologies (Cohen et al. 2002). **(pp. 216–221)**

11.4 Which of the following dementias is characterized by prominent early changes in behavior, personality, or language, as opposed to impairments in memory and other aspects of cognition?

   A. Alzheimer's disease.
   B. Frontotemporal lobar dementia.
   C. Lewy body dementia.
   D. Parkinson's disease dementia.
   E. Vascular dementia.

The correct response is option B.

In FTLD typically there are prominent early changes in behavior, personality, or language as opposed to impairments in memory and other aspects of cognition. As a consequence of impaired judgment and social inappropriateness, patients may have tremendous difficulties in their everyday lives, but on formal psychometric screening they may score entirely within normal limits. **(p. 219)**

11.5 PDD and DLB may be distinguished from Alzheimer's disease by which of the following symptoms that normally occur early on in both PDD and DLB?

   A. Selective recent memory disturbance.
   B. Expressive language defects.
   C. Semantic knowledge impairments.
   D. Impaired judgment.
   E. Visual spatial disturbances.

The correct response is option E.

Both PDD and DLB are characterized by a pattern of memory retrieval problems and mild dysexecutive disturbances, which early in the course are less dramatic and globally impairing than the cognitive deficits of Alzheimer's disease (Hamilton et al. 2004). Visuospatial disturbances are commonly observed early in the course of the Lewy body dementias (Ballard et al. 1999; Hansen et al. 1990; Salmon et al. 1996), but expressive language such as naming tends to be better preserved than in Alzheimer's disease (Ballard et al. 1999; Heyman et al. 1999). Despite these differences on neuropsychological testing, making a solid differential diagnosis based solely on the cognitive profile will be difficult (Monza et al. 1998; Soliveri et al. 2000; Testa et al. 2001). **(p. 221)**

References

Ballard C, Ayre G, O'Brien J: Simple standardized neuropsychological assessment aid in the differential diagnosis of dementia with Lewy bodies and Alzheimer's disease and vascular dementia. Dement Geriatr Cogn Disord 10:104–108, 1999

Bayles KA, Boone DR, Tomoeda CK, et al: Differentiating Alzheimer's patients from the normal elderly and stroke patients with aphasia. J Speech Hear Disord 54:74–87, 1989

Benke T: Two forms of apraxia in Alzheimer's disease. Cortex 29:715–725, 1993

Botwinick J: Intellectual abilities, in The Handbook of the Psychology of Aging. Edited by Birren JE, Schaie KW. New York, Van Nostrand Reinhold, 1977, pp 508–605

Braak H, Braak E: Neuropathological stageing of Alzheimer-related changes. Acta Neuropathol 82:239–259, 1991

Coffey CE, Wilkinson WE, Parashos IA, et al: Quantitative cerebral anatomy of the aging human brain: a cross-sectional study using magnetic resonance imaging. Neurology 43:527–536, 1992

Cohen RA, Paul RH, Ott BR, et al: The relationship of subcortical MRI hyperintensities and brain volume to cognitive function in vascular dementia. J Int Neuropsychol Soc 8:743–752, 2002

Daigneault S, Braun CM: Working memory and the Self-Ordered Pointing Task: further evidence of early prefrontal decline in normal aging. J Clin Exp Neuropsychol 15:881–895, 1993

Finkel D, Reynolds CA, McArdle JJ, et al: Age changes in processing speed as a leading indicator of cognitive aging. Psychol Aging 22:558–568, 2007

Gur RC, Gur RE, Obrist WD, et al: Age and regional cerebral blood flow at rest and during cognitive activity. Arch Gen Psychiatry 44:617–621, 1987

Hamilton JM, Salmon DP, Galasko D, et al: A comparison of episodic memory deficits in neuropathologically confirmed Dementia with Lewy bodies and Alzheimer's disease. J Int Neuropsychol Soc 10:689–697, 2004

Hansen L, Salmon D, Galasko D, et al: The Lewy body variant of Alzheimer's disease: a clinical and pathological entity. Neurology 40:1–8, 1990

Haug H, Barmwater U, Eggers R, et al: Anatomical changes in aging brain: morphometric analysis of the human proscencephalon, in Neuropharmacology, Vol 21: Aging. Edited by Cervos-Navarro J, Sarkander HI. New York, Raven, 1983, pp 1–12

Heyman A, Fillenbaum GG, Gearing M, et al: Comparison of Lewy body variant of Alzheimer's disease with pure Alzheimer's disease: Consortium to Establish a Registry for Alzheimer's Disease, Part XIX. Neurology 52:1839–1844, 1999

Horn J: The theory of fluid and crystallized intelligence in relation to concepts of cognitive psychology and aging in adulthood, in Aging and Cognitive Processes. Edited by Craik F, Trehub S. New York, Plenum, 1982, pp 237–278

Hyman BT, Van Hoesen GW, Damasio AR, et al: Alzheimer's disease: cell-specific pathology isolates the hippocampal formation. Science 225:1168–1170, 1984

Langley LK, Madden DJ: Functional neuroimaging of memory: implications for cognitive aging. Microsc Res Tech 51:75–84, 2000

Locascio JJ, Growdon JH, Corkin S: Cognitive test performance in detecting, staging, and tracking Alzheimer's disease. Arch Neurol 52:1087–1099, 1995

Mickes L, Wixted JT, Fennema-Notestine C, et al: Progressive impairment on neuropsychological tasks in a longitudinal study of preclinical Alzheimer's disease. Neuropsychology 21:696–705, 2007

Mittenberg W, Seidenberg M, O'Leary DS, et al: Changes in cerebral functioning associated with normal aging. J Clin Exp Neuropsychol 11:918–932, 1989

Monza D, Soliveri P, Radice D, et al: Cognitive dysfunction and impaired organization of complex motility in degenerative parkinsonism syndromes. Arch Neurol 55:372–378, 1998

Ratnavalli E, Brayne C, Dawson K, et al: The prevalence of frontotemporal dementia. Neurology 58:1615–1621, 2002

Reid WG, Hely MA, Morris JG, et al: A longitudinal study of Parkinson's disease: clinical and neuropsychological correlates of dementia. J Clin Neurosci 3:327–333, 1996

Salmon DP, Galasko D, Hansen LA, et al: Neuropsychological deficits associated with diffuse Lewy body disease. Brain Cogn 31:148–165, 1996

Salthouse TA: Relations between cognitive abilities and measures of executive functioning. Neuropsychology 19:532–545, 2005

Small BJ, Fratiglioni L, Viitanen M, et al: The course of cognitive impairment in preclinical Alzheimer disease: three- and 6-year follow-up of a population-based sample. Arch Neurol 57:839–844, 2000

Snowden JS, Neary D, Mann DM: Frontotemporal dementia. Br J Psychiatry 180:140–143, 2002

Soliveri P, Monza D, Paridi D, et al: Neuropsychological follow up in patients with Parkinson's disease, striatonigral degeneration type multisystem atrophy and progressive supranuclear palsy. J Neurol Neurosurg Psychiatry 69:313–318, 2000

Storandt M, Grant EA, Miller JP, et al: Longitudinal course and neuropathologic outcomes in original vs revised MCI and in pre-MCI. Neurology 67:467–473, 2006

Testa D, Monza D, Ferrarini M, et al: Comparison of natural histories of progressive supranuclear palsy and multiple system atrophy. Neurol Sci 22:247–251, 2001

Tierney MC, Black SE, Szalai JP, et al: Recognition memory and verbal fluency differentiate probable Alzheimer disease from subcortical ischemic vascular dementia. Arch Neurol 58:1654–1659, 2001

Tisserand DJ: Structural and Functional Changes Underlying Cognitive Aging. Maastricht, The Netherlands, Maastricht University, 2003

Van Gorp WG, Mahler ME: Subcortical features of normal aging, in Subcortical Dementia. Edited by Cummings JL. New York, Oxford University Press, 1990, pp 231–250

Welsh KA, Butters N, Hughes JP, et al: Detection and staging of dementia in Alzheimer's disease: use of the neuropsychological measures developed for the Consortium to Establish a Registry for Alzheimer's Disease (CERAD). Arch Neurol 49:448–452, 1992

Williams-Gray CH, Foltynie T, Brayne CE, et al: Evolution of cognitive dysfunction in an incident Parkinson's disease cohort. Brain 130 (pt 7):1787–1798, 2007

Chapter 12

Delirium

Select the single best response for each question.

12.1 Key clinical features of delirium that are assessed by the Confusion Assessment Method (CAM) include all of the following *except*

A. Inattention.
B. Stable course.
C. Acute onset.
D. Disorganized thinking.
E. Altered level of consciousness.

The correct response is option B.

The CAM (Inouye et al. 1990) provides a simple diagnostic algorithm that has become widely used as a practical means for identification of delirium. The CAM diagnosis of delirium is based on an assessment of the clinical features of 1) acute onset and fluctuating course, 2) inattention, 3) disorganized thinking, and 4) altered level of consciousness. Sudden and acute onset, alteration in attention, and fluctuating course are the central features of delirium. Therefore, it is important to establish a patient's level of baseline cognitive functioning and the course of cognitive change when evaluating for the presence of delirium. A detailed and in-depth background interview with a proxy informant, such as a family member, caregiver, or medical professional who knows the patient, proves invaluable when documenting change in a patient's mental status. It is important to differentiate between 1) cognitive changes that increase and decrease in severity over a period of days, indicative of delirium, and 2) changes that are more chronic and progressive over a period of months to years, indicative of dementia. To fulfill the criteria for delirium, the change in cognitive status must occur in the context of a medical illness, a metabolic disorder, drug toxicity, or drug withdrawal. **(pp. 229–230)**

12.2 Several neurotransmitters have been implicated in the mechanism of delirium. The most frequently considered neurotransmitter for which there is the most evidence is

A. Acetylcholine.
B. Norepinephrine.
C. Glutamate.
D. Melatonin.
E. Dopamine.

The correct response is option A.

The most frequently considered mechanism of delirium is dysfunction in the cholinergic system. Acetylcholine plays a key role in mediating consciousness and attentional process. Given that delirium is manifested by an acute confusional state, often with alterations of consciousness, it is likely to have a cholinergic basis. Evidence for the cholinergic connection includes findings that anticholinergic drugs can induce delirium in humans and animals and that serum anticholinergic activity is increased in patients with delirium (Marcantonio et al. 2006).

Also, cholinesterase inhibitors have been found to reduce symptoms of delirium in some studies (Gleason 2003; Wengel et al. 1998). An excess of dopaminergic neurotransmitters has also been cited as a mechanism of delirium and is most likely related to the role it plays in regulating the release of acetylcholine (Trzepacz and van der Mast 2002). Elevated serotonin, such as that seen in hepatic encephalopathy and "serotonin syndrome," is another proposed mechanism of delirium (Marcantonio et al. 2006).

Other neurotransmitters, including norepinephrine, glutamate, and melatonin, have also been implicated in the development of delirium, most likely due to their interactions with cholinergic and dopaminergic pathways; however, support for their involvement is less substantiated (Cole 2004; Inouye 2006). (pp. 231–232)

12.3 Which of the following is the leading risk factor for development of delirium?

    A. Advanced age.
    B. Male gender.
    C. Vision or hearing impairments.
    D. Alcohol abuse or dependence.
    E. Dementia.

The correct response is option E.

Existing cognitive impairment and dementia are the leading risk factors for the development of delirium (Inouye 2006). In fact, patients with dementia have a two- to fivefold increased risk for developing delirium, and nearly two-thirds of cases of delirium occur in patients with dementia (Cole 2004; Inouye 2006; Trzepacz and van der Mast 2002). Other predisposing factors include advanced age, chronic or severe underlying illness, number and severity of comorbid conditions, functional impairment, male gender, dehydration, vision or hearing impairments, chronic renal insufficiency, history of alcohol abuse or dependence, and malnutrition (Elie et al. 1998; Francis 1992; Rockwood 1989; Rogers et al. 1989). (p. 233)

12.4 A predictive risk model that identifies predisposing factors for delirium has been developed for hospitalized older patients at discharge. Which of the following is *not* one of these risk factors?

    A. Use of physical restraints during delirium.
    B. Functional impairment.
    C. High comorbidity.
    D. Auditory impairment.
    E. Dementia.

The correct response is option D.

Predictive risk models that identify predisposing factors for delirium have been developed in specific medical populations, such as surgical patients, cancer patients, and nursing home patients (Boyle 2006; Hamann et al. 2005). A validated model for prediction of persistent delirium in hospitalized older patients at discharge has identified five risk factors: dementia, vision impairment, functional impairment, high comorbidity, and use of physical restraints during delirium (Inouye et al. 2007). Overall, the development of these risk models aids in understanding the contribution of patient characteristics to delirium risk. (pp. 233–234)

12.5 The key diagnostic feature(s) present in delirium but not dementia is/are

    A. Visual hallucinations.
    B. Cognitive impairment.
    C. Acute onset.
    D. Memory disturbance.
    E. Delusions.

The correct response is option C.

The key diagnostic feature that aids in distinguishing these two conditions is that delirium has an acute and rapid onset, whereas dementia is much more gradual in progression. Alterations in attention and changes in level of consciousness also point to a diagnosis of delirium. However, establishing the occurrence of those changes can be difficult if baseline cognitive data are missing or if preexisting cognitive deficits are reported by an informant. If the differentiation cannot be made with certainty, then given the life-threatening nature of delirium, the patient should be treated as delirious until proven otherwise. **(p. 236)**

12.6 First-line nonpharmacological treatment approaches to delirium should *not* include

    A. Frequent eye contact.
    B. Clear instructions.
    C. Assessment and correction of sensory deficits.
    D. Verbal reorienting strategies.
    E. Use of physical restraints.

The correct response is option E.

In general, nonpharmacological approaches should be implemented as the first-line treatment of delirium. Nonpharmacological treatment approaches include reorientation (e.g., using orientation boards, clocks, calendars), behavioral interventions, encouraging the presence of family members, and transferring a disruptive patient to a private room or closer to the nurse's station for increased supervision. Consistent and compassionate staff are essential in facilitating contact and communication with the patient through frequent verbal reorienting strategies, clear instructions, frequent eye contact, and the inclusion of patients as much as possible in all decision making regarding their daily and medical care. Sensory deficits should be assessed and then corrected by ensuring that all assistive devices, such as eyeglasses and hearing aids, are readily available, functioning, and being used properly by the patient. The use of physical restraints should be minimized due to their role in prolonging delirium, worsening agitation, and increasing complications such as strangulation (Inouye et al. 2007). Strategies that increase the patient's mobility, self-care, and independence should be promoted. Other environmental interventions include limiting room and staff changes, as well as providing a quiet patient care setting with low-level lighting at night, allowing for an uninterrupted period for sleep.

If required, neuroleptics are the first line of pharmacological treatment. Haloperidol is the most widely used agent, with documented efficacy to decrease agitation associated with delirium (Breitbart et al. 1996). Atypical antipsychotics that have been used in the treatment of delirium include risperidone, olanzapine, and quetiapine; however, these agents have been tested in only small, uncontrolled studies and may be associated with a higher mortality rate among older patients with dementia (Inouye 2006). Benzodiazepines typically lead to oversedation and exacerbation of confusion and are therefore not recommended in treating most forms of delirium (Breitbart et al. 1996); however, benzodiazepines still remain the treatment of choice in treating alcohol or sedative-hypnotic drug withdrawal symptoms. For geriatric patients, lorazepam is the preferred agent for treating these symptoms because of its shorter half-life, lack of active metabolites, and availability in parenteral form. **(pp. 237, 239)**

References

Boyle DA: Delirium in older adults with cancer: implications for practice and research. Oncol Nurs Forum 33:61–78, 2006

Breitbart W, Marotta R, Platt MM, et al: A double-blind trial of haloperidol, chlorpromazine, and lorazepam in the treatment of delirium in hospitalized AIDS patients. Am J Psychiatry 153:231–237, 1996

Cole MG: Delirium in elderly patients. Am J Geriatr Psychiatry 12:7–21, 2004

Elie M, Cole MG, Primeau FJ, et al: Delirium risk factors in elderly hospitalized patients. J Gen Intern Med 13:204–212, 1998

Francis J: Delirium in older patients. J Am Geriatr Soc 40:829–838, 1992

Gleason OC: Donepezil for postoperative delirium. Psychosomatics 44:437–438, 2003

Hamann J, Bickel H, Schwaibold H, et al: Postoperative acute confusional state in typical urologic population: incidence, risk factors, and strategies for prevention. Urology 65:449–453, 2005

Inouye SK: Current concepts: delirium in older persons. N Engl J Med 354:1157–1165, 2006

Inouye SK, van Dyck CH, Alessi CA, et al: Clarifying confusion: the Confusion Assessment Method—a new method for detection of delirium. Ann Intern Med 113:941–948, 1990

Inouye SK, Zhang Y, Jones RN, et al: Risk factors for delirium at discharge: development and validation of a predictive model. Arch Intern Med 167:1406–1413, 2007

Marcantonio ER, Rudolph JL, Culley D, et al: Serum biomarkers for delirium. J Gerontol A Biol Sci Med Sci 61:1281–1286, 2006

Rockwood K: Acute confusion in elderly medical patients. J Am Geriatr Soc 37:150–154, 1989

Rogers MP, Liang MH, Daltroy LH, et al: Delirium after elective orthopedic surgery: risk factors and natural history. Int J Psychiatry Med 19:109–121, 1989

Trzepacz PT, van der Mast R: The neuropathophysiology of delirium, in Delirium in Old Age. Edited by Lindesay J, Rockwood K, MacDonald AJ. New York, Oxford University Press, 2002, pp 51–90

Wengel SP, Roccaforte WH, Burke WJ: Donepezil improves symptoms of delirium in dementia: implications for future research. J Geriatr Psychiatry Neurol 11:159–161, 1998

Chapter 13

Dementia and Milder Cognitive Syndromes

Select the single best response for each question.

13.1 You have a 65-year-old patient who presents with a clinical syndrome consisting of a measurable decline in memory with little effect on day-to-day functioning. Which of the following best describes this syndrome?

 A. Delirium.
 B. Dementia.
 C. Alzheimer's disease.
 D. Cognitive impairment not dementia (CIND).
 E. Mild cognitive impairment (MCI).

The correct response is option D.

CIND is a clinical syndrome consisting of a measurable or evident decline in memory or other cognitive abilities, with little effect on day-to-day functioning.
Dementia is a clinical syndrome not entirely caused by delirium, consisting of global cognitive decline, with memory plus one other area of cognition affected, and significant effect on day-to-day functioning.
Alzheimer's disease is a brain disease characterized by plaques, tangles, and neuronal loss.
MCI is a clinical syndrome that is a subgroup of CIND and most likely is the prodrome to Alzheimer's dementia. It can be amnestic (having memory deficits) or nonamnestic. **(p. 244)**

13.2 For the dementia syndrome to be present, key elements must be exhibited by the patient. Which of the following is *not* one of these key elements?

 A. Basic daily living activities must be impaired.
 B. The cognitive symptoms must represent a cognitive decline.
 C. The cognitive syndrome must be present in the absence of delirium.
 D. The person's daily functioning must be impaired.
 E. Only one area of cognition may be affected.

The correct response is option E.

For the dementia syndrome to be present, several areas of cognition must be affected (*global*). To differentiate dementia from mental retardation, the cognitive symptoms must represent a cognitive *decline* for the individual. The decline must be significant, typically sufficient to affect the person's daily functioning (operationalized as instrumental or basic daily living activities). Finally, because delirium can cause the full range of cognitive symptoms associated with dementia, it is critical that the cognitive syndrome be present in the *absence of delirium*. This broad definition has been operationalized in several criteria, with those of DSM-IV-TR (American Psychiatric Association 2000) being the most commonly used. **(p. 244)**

13.3 Traditionally, dementia is differentiated into cortical and subcortical subsyndromes. Which of the following areas of impairment is indicative of subcortical dementia?

    A. Amnesia.
    B. Apraxia.
    C. Dysexecutive.
    D. Aphasia.
    E. Agnosia.

The correct response is option C.

The cortical subsyndrome refers to losses of cognitive *abilities*, whereas the subcortical subsyndrome refers to losses in the *coordination* of these abilities—sometimes referred to as executive functioning or executive control. The cortical subsyndrome is characterized by the four A's of impairment (amnesia, apraxia, aphasia, agnosia), and the subcortical subsyndrome by the four D's (dysmnesia, delay, dysexecutive symptoms, depletion). **(p. 244)**

13.4 Which of the following neuropsychiatric symptom clusters is indicative of loss of executive control?

    A. Spontaneous violence, intrusions, wandering.
    B. Sleep, sexual, or feeding disturbances.
    C. Delusions and hallucinations.
    D. Apathy, depression, anxiety, and irritability.
    E. None of the above.

The correct response is option A.

Dementia has been associated with several neuropsychiatric symptoms. These are generally grouped into four types: 1) affective and motivational symptoms, such as apathy, depression, anxiety, and irritability; 2) perceptual disturbances, such as delusions and hallucinations; 3) disturbances of basic drives, including sleep, sexuality, and feeding; and 4) disturbances typically arising in more severe dementia, representing unexpected, socially inappropriate, or disinhibited behaviors. These inappropriate behaviors, which include spontaneous violence, intrusiveness, wandering, and the like, represent behavioral manifestations of loss of executive control, sometimes referred to as executive dysfunction syndrome (Lyketsos et al. 2004). **(pp. 244–245)**

13.5 The Mini-Mental State Examination (MMSE) is widely used as a screening instrument for dementia. What is its major limitation?

    A. It must be administered by individuals skilled in its use.
    B. It is unable to detect severe forms of dementia.
    C. It is time-consuming to administer.
    D. It has limitations in evaluating executive control function.
    E. It does not provide a numerical score.

The correct response is option D.

Conducting a cognitive assessment is the central aspect of the evaluation. Many specialists tend to use the Mini-Mental State Examination (Folstein et al. 1975) as their primary tool. The MMSE may be appropriate in more severe dementia but is inefficient in evaluating patients with milder cognitive symptoms or mild dementia because the MMSE has ceiling effects, especially for premorbidly well-educated and intelligent individuals, and has limitations in evaluating executive control function. Specialists in geriatric psychiatry and other clinicians who work with patients who have dementia will need to broaden their bedside standardized assessments. The Modified Mini-Mental State (3MS) provides a broader assessment of cognition (Teng and Chui 1987). The 3MS has many advantages: several translations exist; it has been validated in Spanish, Chinese, and other languages; it assesses abstract thinking, delayed recall, and verbal fluency better than the MMSE; and it has well-known population norms. **(p. 246)**

13.6   Which of the following dementia syndromes is the second most common form of dementia in persons under age 65, with a rate of occurrence that is close to that of Alzheimer's disease?

   A. Parkinson's disease dementia (PDD).
   B. Frontotemporal degeneration (FTD).
   C. Dementia with Lewy bodies (DLB).
   D. Dementia due to normal pressure hydrocephalus.
   E. Dementia due to prion diseases.

The correct response is option B.

FTD is in many ways the paradigmatic non-Alzheimer's dementia and has recently become a major focus of interest because of the appreciation that in individuals under age 65, FTD is the second most common form of dementia, with a rate of occurrence that is close to that of Alzheimer's dementia (Neary et al. 2005). Previously referred to as Pick's disease, FTD is heterogeneous both clinically and pathologically (Kertesz 2005; Neary et al. 2005). The clinical syndrome typically begins with changes in behavior, affect, and personality, which result in disinhibition, hyperorality, social inappropriateness, apathy, and related symptoms of loss of executive control.

   Patients with PDD typically show impairments in executive functioning, including delays in problem solving, difficulties in set shifting, and poor fluency. They also have memory impairments characteristic of dysmnesia, affecting working memory and the organization of explicit memory. Some have visuospatial difficulties arising out of difficulty with set shifting and the need for high executive demand to complete visuospatial tests. In early to mid-stage Parkinson's disease, 16%–20% of patients develop dementia, in contrast to as many as 80% in later Parkinson's disease.

   The central feature of DLB is a progressive dementia with primary persistent memory impairment and deficits in attention, executive, and visuospatial abilities. Core features, at least one of which is necessary for the diagnosis of DLB, include fluctuating cognition with pronounced variations in attention and alertness, visual hallucinations, and spontaneous parkinsonism.

   The dementia of normal pressure hydrocephalus is a subcortical dementia associated with a characteristic magnetic-like gait disorder and incontinence.

   Recent knowledge regarding prion protein transmission across species has led to concerns about animal-to-human transmission of these proteins through the diet, followed by incurable, rapidly progressive dementias. The annual incidence of Creutzfeldt-Jakob dementia is on the order of 1 per million per year worldwide, with a few hundred cases presenting every year in the United States (Caramelli et al. 2006). **(pp. 250–253)**

13.7   Which of the following cholinesterase inhibitors is available in patch form and has been approved by the U.S. Food and Drug Administration (FDA) to treat PDD?

   A. Huperzine.
   B. Tacrine.
   C. Donepezil.
   D. Galantamine.
   E. Rivastigmine.

The correct response is option E.

The cholinesterase inhibitors huperzine, tacrine, donepezil, rivastigmine, and galantamine are all approved by the FDA or otherwise available in the United States for treatment of the cognitive symptoms of Alzheimer's dementia. Most of these medications have been approved for the treatment of mild to moderate Alzheimer's dementia; donepezil has been approved for the treatment of severe Alzheimer's dementia. They are available in a variety of formulations as pills, as delayed-release pills, and in patch form (rivastigmine only). Huperzine, an over-the-counter nutraceutical that is currently under study and whose safety is poorly known, and tacrine, which has hepatotoxicity concerns, are used very infrequently. Although clinical trials have suggested that cholinesterase inhibitors may be of value in treating vascular dementia, none of them has been approved by the FDA for that purpose. The results of one study suggest that donepezil is associated with increased mortality in vascular dementia relative to placebo. Rivastigmine has been approved for the treatment of Parkinson's disease dementia and has also been found in randomized trials to be effective in dementia with Lewy bodies. **(p. 254)**

References

American Psychiatric Association: Diagnostic and Statistical Manual of Mental Disorders, 4th Edition, Text Revision. Washington, DC, American Psychiatric Association, 2000

Caramelli M, Ru G, Acutis P, et al: Prion diseases: current understanding of epidemiology and pathogenesis, and therapeutic advances. CNS Drugs 20:15–28, 2006

Folstein MF, Folstein SE, McHugh PR: "Mini-mental state": a practical method for grading the cognitive state of patients for the clinician. J Psychiatr Res 12:189–198, 1975

Lyketsos CG, Rosenblatt A, Rabins P: Forgotten frontal lobe syndrome or "executive dysfunction syndrome." Psychosomatics 45:247–255, 2004

Kertesz A: Frontotemporal dementia: one disease, or many? Probably one, possibly two. Alzheimer Dis Assoc Disord 19 (suppl 1):S19–S24, 2005

Neary D, Snowden J, Mann D: Frontotemporal dementia. Lancet Neurol 4:771–780, 2005

Teng EL, Chui HC: The Modified Mini-Mental State (3MS) examination. J Clin Psychiatry 48:314–318, 1987

Chapter 14

Movement Disorders

Select the single best response for each question.

14.1 Parkinsonism has been associated with the use of antipsychotic medications. Which of the following agents is *least* likely to produce parkinsonism symptoms?

    A. Haloperidol.
    B. Olanzapine.
    C. Quetiapine.
    D. Risperidone.
    E. Thioridazine.

The correct response is option C.

Parkinsonism is well known to be associated with use of dopamine receptor–blocking agents, including antipsychotic medications and antiemetics. Classic antipsychotic medications typically exhibit strong antagonism at dopamine D_2 receptors (Mendis et al. 1994), whereas the newer atypical antipsychotics have less affinity for dopamine D_2 receptors. The newer agents have fewer parkinsonian side effects but are not totally free of them (Chouinard et al. 1993). Based on clinical experience with patients with Parkinson's disease who have levodopa-related psychosis, among the newer agents risperidone has the greatest number of parkinsonian side effects, followed by olanzapine and then quetiapine. Clozapine exhibits a lower relative affinity for dopamine D_2 receptors compared with conventional antipsychotics (Meltzer 1992) and suppresses levodopa-related psychosis in Parkinson's disease while minimizing exacerbation of Parkinson's disease symptoms; however, clozapine can suppress bone marrow, and thus blood counts must be monitored. **(pp. 261–262)**

14.2 Parkinson's disease is a chronic, progressive, neurodegenerative illness that produces a constellation of motoric symptoms. Which of the following symptoms usually does *not* occur in Parkinson's disease?

    A. Rigidity.
    B. Bradykinesia.
    C. Postural instability.
    D. Intention tremor.
    E. Hypomimia.

The correct response is option D.

Parkinson's disease is a chronic, progressive, neurodegenerative illness that produces rigidity, slowness of movement (bradykinesia), postural instability, and, often, tremor at rest. Other common clinical features of Parkinson's disease include hypomimia (masked facies or facial masking), micrographia (small handwriting), stooped posture, retropulsion, and shuffling and festinating gait. **(p. 262)**

14.3 There are a number of motor complications of Parkinson's disease. Which of the following symptoms is usually secondary to medications used to treat Parkinson's disease?

    A. Retropulsion.
    B. On-off phenomena.
    C. Postural instability.
    D. Freezing of gait.
    E. Festination.

The correct response is option B.

Motor complications that occur in Parkinson's disease as the disease progresses are medication-related dyskinesias (involuntary writhing, twisting, and/or head bobbing movements associated with levodopa replacement therapy), motor fluctuations, and on-off phenomena in which the patient experiences "on" time when medications are working and the patient can move better but experiences "off" times when medication effects wear off (Pahwa et al. 2006).

Postural instability usually occurs later than other clinical signs of Parkinson's disease and can be very disabling. Patients fall because of an inability to keep their feet under their center of gravity, and these patients exhibit retropulsion (inability to maintain balance when suddenly displaced backward) and anteropulsion (inability to maintain balance when suddenly displaced forward). Freezing of gait occurs when the feet appear to become stuck to the floor during attempted walking. Sometimes, a patient can overcome this freezing by performing a motor trick such as kicking his or her walking cane to initiate gait. Festination occurs in an upright, walking patient with Parkinson's disease whose feet are lagging behind his or her center of gravity. This clinical sign manifests as rapid, tiny steps taken to keep from falling. **(p. 263)**

14.4 You have a 72-year-old male patient who currently is on no medications and was recently diagnosed with Parkinson's disease by a neurologist. The most effective pharmacologic treatment is the administration of which of the following classes of medications?

    A. Anticholinergic agent.
    B. Monoamine oxidase B inhibitor.
    C. Dopamine agonist.
    D. Catechol O-methyltransferase (COMT) inhibitor.
    E. Dopamine precursor.

The correct response is option E.

Parkinson's disease results from a deficiency of the neurotransmitter dopamine in the brain, and administration of levodopa, a precursor of dopamine, is the most effective treatment for Parkinson's disease symptoms.

Anticholinergic medications (trihexyphenidyl, benztropine) are sometimes used to treat early Parkinson's disease symptoms. Amantadine, an antiviral medication with anticholinergic and antiglutamate effects, produces mild improvement of parkinsonism early in the disease course, in part because of enhanced release of endogenous dopamine stores from the substantia nigra.

Selegiline is a relatively selective monoamine oxidase B inhibitor that delays the need for therapeutic treatment with levodopa in early Parkinson's disease by several months. However, selegiline's modest effect on parkinsonian symptoms appears to be due to the drug's metabolism to an amphetamine-like metabolite that blocks synaptic dopamine reuptake, rather than to a true neuroprotective effect.

Dopamine agonists are useful adjuncts in the symptomatic treatment of Parkinson's disease. These agents act directly on dopamine receptors and are particularly useful in smoothing the therapeutic response to levodopa by reducing motor fluctuations ("on-off" phenomena) and by increasing the period of benefit obtained from each dose of levodopa.

Entacapone and tolcapone are COMT inhibitors that reduce the breakdown of levodopa before it reaches the brain. Some COMT inhibitors may also slow the breakdown of dopamine in the brain. Because of rare, fulminant hepatotoxicity, tolcapone is not much used clinically. **(p. 264)**

14.5 Which of the following movement disorders produces myoclonic, apraxic, rigid, akinetic movements and alien hand syndrome, in which one hand seems to have a mind of its own?

    A. Cortical-basal ganglionic degeneration (CBGD).
    B. Frontotemporal dementia.
    C. Multiple system atrophy.
    D. Progressive supranuclear palsy.
    E. Normal pressure hydrocephalus.

The correct response is option A.

CBGD, also referred to as corticobasal degeneration, causes marked, asymmetric parkinsonism and dystonia (Litvan et al. 1997; Riley and Lang 2000; Schneider et al. 1997). Resting tremor is uncommon in this condition. CBGD can result in jerky (myoclonic), apraxic, rigid, akinetic movements and alien hand syndrome. There may be early dementia, cortical sensory findings (such as hemineglect to double simultaneous tactile stimulation), and unilateral agraphesthesia (manifested as the inability to identify a number written on the palm of one's hand). Stimulus-sensitive myoclonus and action tremor may also occur.

In the degenerative condition of frontotemporal dementia and parkinsonism linked to chromosome 17 (FTDP-17), insidious onset of behavioral and motor changes occurs. Cognitive impairment typically leads to dementia, parkinsonism, nonfluent aphasia, a change in personality, and/or psychosis (Foster et al. 1997; Lund and Manchester Groups 1994). Onset is generally in the fifth decade of life and can be as late as the sixth decade.

Multiple system atrophy (MSA) encompasses several "Parkinson's plus" conditions that are characterized by bilateral, symmetric parkinsonism that is poorly responsive to levodopa therapy, as well as the absence or near absence of tremor (Quinn 1994; Shulman and Weiner 1997; Wenning et al. 1994). MSA can be divided into three main clinical types: MSA-parkinsonism (MSA-P), in which parkinsonism is the main clinical feature; MSA-cerebellar (MSA-C), in which cerebellar ataxia is the main clinical feature; and MSA-autonomic (MSA-A), in which autonomic dysfunction such as severe orthostatic hypotension is a major clinical feature. MSA-P represents a majority of cases.

Progressive supranuclear palsy (PSP), or Steele-Richardson-Olszewski syndrome, is a progressive, neurodegenerative condition consisting of parkinsonism without prominent tremor, vertical gaze palsy, axial (midline) more than appendicular (arm and leg) rigidity, early postural instability, and poor response to levodopa (Golbe and Davis 1993; Litvan 1998; Litvan et al. 1996). The syndrome was first described by Steele et al. (1964). The Society for Progressive Supranuclear Palsy estimates that 20,000 people in the United States have PSP—only 3,000–4,000 of whom have received a diagnosis—yielding an estimated known prevalence in the United States of 1.39 per 100,000. PSP is often associated with frequent falling, lack of eye contact, monotonous speech, sloppy eating, and slowed mentation (Jankovic et al. 1990).

Normal pressure hydrocephalus (NPH), also known as communicating hydrocephalus, is more common in elderly persons than in younger adults and can result in a progressive gait disorder, urinary incontinence, and memory decline. It can be caused by slowed flow of cerebrospinal fluid (CSF) across the arachnoid villi and out of the brain via the superior sagittal sinus. NPH can develop after meningitis or a subarachnoid bleed but more commonly develops in the absence of these relatively rare conditions. Individuals with NPH may take small steps and exhibit a "magnetic gait," in which they experience difficulty lifting their feet to walk because of a sense that their feet are stuck to the ground. The triad of gait disorder, urinary incontinence, and memory loss suggests a diagnosis of NPH. **(pp. 266–268)**

14.6 There are a number of hyperkinetic movement disorders. Which of the following consists of rhythmic oscillations across a joint resulting from involuntary, alternating activation of agonist and antagonist muscles?

    A. Chorea.
    B. Dystonia.
    C. Essential tremor.
    D. Myoclonus.
    E. Tics.

The correct response is option C.

Tremor consists of rhythmic oscillations across a joint resulting from involuntary, alternating activation of agonist and antagonist muscles. For example, wrist tremor is caused by alternating activation and relaxation of forearm flexor and extensor muscles. Essential tremor is the most prevalent movement disorder among adults, affecting up to 2% of the general population. The prevalence of essential tremor increases with age; estimates range up to more than 10% in individuals older than age 70 years. Also called *benign essential tremor* and *familial tremor*, essential tremor may not be benign and can result in severe impairment in activities of daily living in some individuals. Essential tremor manifests as postural and kinetic tremor at the arms and hands; the head and voice are often involved (Benito-Leon and Louis 2007).

Chorea is characterized by involuntary, dancelike movements that consist of continuous, random, unpredictable, often twitchlike motions that flow from one body part to another. Chorea can be hard to distinguish from tardive dyskinesia in the absence of a complete history; however, movements in chorea are more random, and movements in tardive dyskinesia tend to be repetitive and stereotyped.

Dystonia is a movement disorder that usually begins by middle age and may persist in elderly individuals (Scott 2000; Tarsy and Simon 2006). In dystonia, involuntary muscle spasms result in bizarre, sustained postures. These postures initially occur during attempted voluntary movement and may persist at rest. Dystonia can be idiopathic (associated with no identifiable structural abnormality) or secondary (associated with a known structural lesion demonstrated by an imaging study) and can have delayed onset, appearing after a previous injury (Scott and Jankovic 1996).

Myoclonus refers to sudden jerklike or shocklike movements caused by involuntary activation of affected muscles (positive myoclonus) or to sudden loss of activation of affected muscles (negative myoclonus) (Vercueil 2006). The movements can occur randomly or with regular frequency. Myoclonus can arise from dysfunction at multiple levels of the central nervous system, from cortex to brain stem to spinal cord.

Tics are brief, repetitive, semi-voluntary, jerklike movements. Vocal tics consist of audible vocalizations, and motor tics consist of rapid movements of the head, face, limbs, and other body parts. Tics can be simple or complex. They can usually be suppressed for a short time. During voluntary suppression of tics, patients may feel unpleasant sensations building up in an involved body part and experience transient relief from the unpleasant sensation by performing the tic once again. Tourette's syndrome, a tic disorder that begins in childhood but can persist in adults (Sheppard et al. 1999), is often associated with obsessive-compulsive disorder, a condition that can become more disabling than the tics themselves. **(pp. 268–270)**

References

Benito-Leon J, Louis ED: Clinical update: diagnosis and treatment of essential tremor. Lancet 369:1152–1154, 2007

Chouinard G, Jones B, Remington G, et al: A Canadian multicenter placebo-controlled study of fixed doses of risperidone and haloperidol in the treatment of chronic schizophrenic patients. J Clin Psychopharmacol 13:25–40, 1993

Foster NL, Wilhelmsen K, Sima AA, et al: Frontotemporal dementia and parkinsonism linked to chromosome 17: a consensus conference. Participants of the Chromosome 17–Related Dementia Conference. Ann Neurol 41:706–715, 1997

Golbe LI, Davis PH: Progressive supranuclear palsy, in Parkinson's Disease and Movement Disorders, 2nd Edition. Edited by Jankovic J, Tolosa E. Baltimore, MD, Williams & Wilkins, 1993, pp 145–161

Jankovic J, Friedman DI, Pirozzolo FJ, et al: Progressive supranuclear palsy: motor, neurobehavioral, and neuro-ophthalmic findings. Adv Neurol 53:293–304, 1990

Litvan I: Progressive supranuclear palsy revisited. Acta Neurol Scand 98:73–84, 1998

Litvan I, Agid Y, Calne D, et al: Clinical research criteria for the diagnosis of progressive supranuclear palsy (Steele-Richardson-Olszewski syndrome): report of the NINDS-SPSP international workshop. Neurology 47:1–9, 1996

Litvan I, Agid Y, Goetz C, et al: Accuracy of the clinical diagnosis of corticobasal degeneration: a clinicopathologic study. Neurology 48:119–125, 1997

Lund and Manchester Groups: Clinical and neuropathological criteria for frontotemporal dementia. J Neurol Neurosurg Psychiatry 57:416–418, 1994

Meltzer HY: The mechanism of action of clozapine in relation to its clinical advantages, in Novel Antipsychotic Drugs. Edited by Meltzer HY. New York, Raven, 1992, pp 1–13

Mendis T, Mohr E, George A, et al: Symptomatic relief from treatment-induced psychosis in Parkinson's disease: an open-label pilot study with remoxipride. Mov Disord 9:197–200, 1994

Pahwa R, Factor SA, Lyons KE, et al: Practice parameter: treatment of Parkinson disease with motor fluctuations and dyskinesia (an evidence-based review). Neurology 66:983–995, 2006

Quinn NP: Multiple system atrophy, in Movement Disorders 3 (Butterworth-Heinemann International Medical Reviews. Neurology 12). Edited by Marsden CD, Fahn S. Boston, MA, Butterworth-Heinemann, 1994, pp 262–281

Riley DE, Lang AE: Clinical diagnostic criteria, in Corticobasal Degeneration (Advances in Neurology, Vol 82). Edited by Litvan I, Goetz CG, Lang AE. Philadelphia, PA, Lippincott Williams & Wilkins, 2000, pp 29–34

Schneider JA, Watts RL, Gearing M, et al: Corticobasal degeneration: neuropathologic and clinical heterogeneity. Neurology 48:959–969, 1997

Scott BL: Evaluation and treatment of dystonia. South Med J 93:746–751, 2000

Scott BL, Jankovic J: Delayed-onset progressive movement disorders after static brain lesions. Neurology 46:68–74, 1996

Sheppard DM, Bradshaw JL, Purcell R, et al: Tourette's and comorbid syndromes: obsessive compulsive and attention deficit hyperactivity disorder: a common etiology? Clin Psychol Rev 19:531–552, 1999

Shulman LM, Weiner WJ: Multiple-system atrophy, in Movement Disorders: Neurologic Principles and Practice. Edited by Watts RL, Koller WC. New York, McGraw-Hill, 1997, pp 297–306

Steele JC, Richardson JC, Olszewski J: Progressive supranuclear palsy: a heterogeneous degeneration involving the brain stem, basal ganglia and cerebellum, with vertical gaze and pseudobulbar palsy, nuchal dystonia and dementia. Arch Neurol 10:333–359, 1964

Tarsy D, Simon DK: Dystonia. N Engl J Med 355:818–829, 2006

Vercueil L: Myoclonus and movement disorders. Neurophysiol Clin 36:327–331, 2006

Wenning GK, Ben Shlomo Y, Magalhaes M, et al: Clinical features and natural history of multiple system atrophy: an analysis of 100 cases. Brain 117:835–845, 1994

C h a p t e r   1 5

Mood Disorders

Select the single best response for each question.

15.1 You diagnose major depression in a physically healthy 76-year-old woman and recommend to her antidepressant medication. She responds by saying, "What's the use? I've heard that antidepressants are not very effective in older people." You state that if seniors are treated with an adequate dose of an antidepressant for a sufficient period of time (at least 6–9 months) they may expect a recovery rate of approximately

  A. 30%.
  B. 40%.
  C. 50%.
  D. 60%.
  E. 70%.

The correct response is option E.

Most clinicians and clinical investigators report that more than 70% of elderly patients with major depression who are treated with antidepressant medication (at an adequate dose for a sufficient time) recover from the index episode of depression if the depression is uncomplicated by comorbid factors. Reynolds et al. (1992) reported that treatment of physically healthy depressed elders with combined interpersonal psychotherapy and nortriptyline was associated with response rates nearing 80%. **(p. 278)**

15.2 Factors associated with improved outcome in late-life depression include which of the following?

  A. Family history of depression.
  B. Male gender.
  C. Introverted personality.
  D. Substance abuse history.
  E. Recent major life events.

The correct response is option A.

Factors associated with improved outcome in late-life depression include a history of recovery from previous episodes, a family history of depression, female gender, extraverted personality, current or recent employment, absence of substance abuse, no history of major psychiatric disorder, less severe depressive symptomatology, and absence of major life events and serious medical illness (Baldwin and Jolley 1986; Cole et al. 1999; Post 1972). **(p. 278)**

15.3 Certain psychological factors may contribute to the onset of late-life depressive symptoms. All of the following factors have been reported by investigators to increase the likelihood or frequency of late-life depressive symptoms *except*

    A. Hopelessness.
    B. Cognitive distortions.
    C. Acceptance.
    D. Higher levels of mastery.
    E. Rumination.

The correct response is option D.

Higher levels of mastery have been shown to have a direct association with fewer depressive symptoms in older adults and to buffer the adverse impact of disability on depression (Jang et al. 2002). Self-efficacy may have a direct effect and also may work indirectly through its effect on social support to prevent depressive symptoms, as indicated in a sample of older adults followed for 1 year (Holahan and Holahan 1987).

In a study comparing older patients with and without personality disorder, specific personality traits were not correlated with clinical features of depression such as age at onset and number of previous episodes, but some of the traits were associated with depressive symptoms such as hopelessness (Morse and Lynch 2004).

Cognitive distortions (Beck 1987) are among the most studied psychological origins of depression across the life cycle. Depressed individuals may overreact to life events or misinterpret these events and exaggerate their adverse outcome.

In a study from a community sample, elderly persons with more frequent depressive symptoms used acceptance, rumination, and catastrophizing (maladaptive cognitive distortions) to a higher extent and positive reappraisal to a lower extent than did those with fewer symptoms (Kraaij and de Wilde 2001). **(pp. 282–283)**

15.4 Adults are thought to acquire increased wisdom as they age. One group of investigators has operationalized wisdom and studied it in community samples. Which of the following criteria is *not* associated with increase wisdom?

    A. Rich factual knowledge.
    B. Absolute values and life priorities.
    C. Life span contextualization.
    D. Recognition and management of uncertainty.
    E. Rich procedural knowledge.

The correct response is option B.

Adults are thought to acquire increased wisdom as they age. Wisdom is a nebulous concept. Investigators with the Berlin Aging Group, however, have operationalized wisdom and studied it in community samples (Baltes and Staudinger 2000). Wisdom is an expert knowledge system concerning the fundamental pragmatics of life, including knowledge and judgment about the meaning and conduct of life and the orchestrating of human development toward excellence while attending conjointly to personal and collective well-being. Five criteria can be used to assess wisdom: rich factual knowledge; rich procedural knowledge (e.g., the ability to develop strategies for addressing problems); life span contextualization (e.g., integrating life experiences); relativism of values and life priorities (e.g., tolerance for differences in society); and recognition and management of uncertainty (accepting that the future cannot be known with certainty and that the ability to assess one's sociocultural environment is inherently constrained). Wisdom is thought to accumulate over the life cycle if severe physical illness and cognitive impairment do not intervene. Cumulative wisdom over time should protect older adults from spiraling down into depression when confronted with a complex of negative experiences. **(pp. 284–285)**

15.5 An investigator compared the clinical, demographic, and social characteristics of psychotic and nonpsychotic depression in a large sample of elderly and younger hospitalized patients and found which of the following variables to be more common in psychotic depression?

    A. Good social support.
    B. Lack of suicidal ideation.
    C. Younger age.
    D. Cerebrovascular risk factors.
    E. Psychomotor agitation.

The correct response is option C.

Thakur et al. (1999) compared the clinical, demographic, and social characteristics of psychotic and nonpsychotic depression in a tertiary care sample of 674 elderly and younger patients. In this study, younger age, psychomotor retardation, guilt, feelings of worthlessness, a history of delusions in the past, and increased suicidal ideation and intent were found more commonly in psychotic than in nonpsychotic patients, and these associations were largely confirmed when sociodemographic variables were controlled. Psychotic depression also tended to be associated with poor social support and, not surprisingly, bipolar illness. Cerebrovascular risk factors did not differ significantly between psychotic and nonpsychotic patients. The weakness of this study is that it dealt with hospitalized patients, not a population-based sample. **(p. 286)**

15.6 Minor, subsyndromal or subthreshold depression is commonly found in the elderly. Associations with subsyndromal depression are similar to those found in major depression, including all of the following *except*

    A. Unmarried status.
    B. Male gender.
    C. Poorer self-rated health.
    D. Perceived low social support.
    E. More disability days.

The correct response is option B.

Associations with subsyndromal depression are similar to those for major depression, including impaired physical functioning, disability days, poorer self-rated health, use of psychotropic medications, perceived low social support, female gender, and unmarried status (Beekman et al. 1995; Hybels et al. 2001). Other investigators have suggested a syndrome of depression without sadness, thought to be more common in older adults (Gallo et al. 1997). **(p. 286)**

References

Baldwin RC, Jolley DJ: The prognosis of depression in old age. Br J Psychiatry 149:574–583, 1986
Baltes P, Staudinger U: Wisdom: a metaheuristic (pragmatic) to orchestrate mind and virtue toward excellence. Am Psychol 55:122–136, 2000
Beck A: Cognitive model of depression. Journal of Cognitive Psychotherapy 1:2–27, 1987
Beekman AT, Deeg DJ, van Tilburg T, et al: Major and minor depression in later life: a study of prevalence and risk factors. J Affect Disord 36:65–75, 1995
Cole MG, Bellavance F, Mansour A: Prognosis of depression in elderly community and primary care populations: a systematic review and meta-analysis. Am J Psychiatry 156:1182–1189, 1999
Gallo JJ, Rabins PV, Lyketsos CG: Depression without sadness: functional outcomes of nondysphoric depression in later life. J Am Geriatr Soc 45:570–578, 1997

Holahan CK, Holahan CJ: Self-efficacy, social support, and depression in aging: a longitudinal analysis. J Gerontol 42:65–68, 1987

Hybels CF, Blazer DG, Pieper CF: Toward a threshold for subthreshold depression: an analysis of correlates of depression by severity of symptoms using data from an elderly community sample. Gerontologist 41:357–365, 2001

Jang Y, Haley WE, Small BJ: The role of mastery and social resources in the associations between disability and depression in later life. Gerontologist 42:80–813, 2002

Kraaij V, de Wilde EJ: Negative life events and depressive symptoms in the elderly: a life span perspective. Aging Ment Health 5:84–91, 2001

Morse JQ, Lynch TR: A preliminary investigation of self-reported personality disorders in late life: prevalence, predictors of depressive severity, and clinical correlates. Aging Ment Health 8:307–315, 2004

Post F: The management and nature of depressive illnesses in late life: a follow-through study. Br J Psychiatry 121:393–404, 1972

Reynolds CF 3rd, Frank E, Perel JM, et al: Combined pharmacotherapy and psychotherapy in the acute and continuation treatment of elderly patients with recurrent major depression: a preliminary report. Am J Psychiatry 149:1687–1692, 1992

Thakur M, Hays J, Krishnan KR: Clinical, demographic, and social characteristics of psychotic depression. Psychiatry Res 86:99–106, 1999

Chapter 16

Bipolar Disorder in Late Life

Select the single best response for each question.

16.1 The exact prevalence of bipolar disorder in late life is uncertain, but several large studies have reported prevalence rates in community samples to be

    A. <0.5%.
    B. 1%–2%.
    C. 3%–5%.
    D. 6%–8%.
    E. 9%–10%.

The correct response is option A.

The exact prevalence of bipolar disorder in late life is uncertain. In the community, the prevalence has generally been reported to range from 0.08% to 0.5% based on four large-scale studies that utilized very different sampling methods. The Epidemiologic Catchment Area study conducted in the early 1990s sampled 18,263 community-dwelling Americans at five sites to determine the prevalence of mental illnesses for those age 15 years or older (Weissman et al. 1988). They found that bipolar disorder for adults age 65 years or older had a 1-year prevalence range of 0–0.5%, with a cross-site mean of 0.1%. This was markedly lower that the prevalence among young (ages 18–44 years; 1.4%) and middle-aged (45–64 years; 0.4%) adults. Similarly, a large HMO administrative database review containing almost 300,000 unique individuals found a prevalence of 0.25% for bipolar disorder in persons age 65 or older, while the prevalence was 0.46% in adults ages 40–64 years (Unutzer et al. 1998). Hirschfeld et al. (2003) sent the Mood Disorder Questionnaire (a validated screening instrument for bipolar I and II disorders) to 127,000 people. In the 85,258 responders, the overall screen rate for bipolar disorder was 3.4%, but for adults age 65 or older, the screen rate was 0.5%. Finally, Klap et al. (2003), conducting a telephone survey of 9,585 households, found a prevalence rate of 0.08% for adults age 65 or older compared with 1.17% for adults ages 30–64. Interestingly, each of these surveys suggested that the prevalence of bipolar disorder declines with age, or in aging cohorts. **(pp. 301–302)**

16.2 Which of the following variables is decreased or lower in older patients with bipolar disorder as compared with younger patients with bipolar disorder?

    A. Depression as the initial episode of illness.
    B. Medical comorbidity.
    C. Substance abuse.
    D. Mortality rates.
    E. Dementia.

The correct response is option C.

Substance abuse, the most common and best-reported comorbid condition in the literature, appears less common in older bipolar patients than in younger bipolar patients; lifetime history of substance abuse also appears less common. Dementia and poorer cognitive performance on neurological testing is possibly increased, or apparent earlier, in older adults with bipolar disorder. Medical comorbidity is also higher in older adults with bipolar disorder (Beyer et al. 2005), with special concern about neurological illness and diabetes. All of these problems may contribute to higher mortality rates in bipolar patients compared with non–psychiatrically ill populations and unipolar depressed patients.

In reviewing studies that retrospectively looked at course prior to hospitalization, Goodwin and Jamison (1990) reported that depression was the initial episode more often in older adults than younger patients. **(p. 304)**

16.3 Evaluation of patients with late-life bipolar disorder reveals various patterns of presentation. Which of the following patterns is the most frequent in elderly patients with bipolar disorder?

A. Those who have never been recognized as having bipolar symptoms or who have been misdiagnosed.
B. Those who previously experienced only episodes of depression but have now switched to a manic episode.
C. Those who have never had bipolar disorder but develop mania due to a specific medical or neurological event.
D. Those who developed bipolar disorder earlier in life and are now seeking treatment.
E. Those who have never had bipolar disorder but develop mania for unknown reasons.

The correct response is option D.

On evaluation, patients with late-life bipolar disorder may present with one of five potential patterns: 1) those who had an early onset of bipolar disease and have now reached old age, 2) those who previously experienced only episodes of depression but have now switched to a manic episode, 3) those who have never had an affective illness, but develop mania due to a specific medical or neurological event (i.e., head trauma, cerebrovascular accident, hyperthyroidism, etc.), 4) those who have never been recognized as having bipolar symptoms or were misdiagnosed, and 5) those who have never had an affective illness but develop mania for unknown reasons. It is unknown how common each presentation may be, although the most frequent experience is encountering a patient who developed bipolar disorder earlier in life and is now seeking treatment. **(p. 308)**

16.4 Hyperintense signals viewed on T2-weighted magnetic resonance imaging (MRI) images are among the earliest and most consistent neuroimaging findings in bipolar disorder. The presence of hyperintensities may be especially important in late-life bipolar disorder. MRI hyperintensities are associated with which of the following?

A. Longer hospital stays and more frequent rehospitalizations.
B. Risk modifiers for cognitive dysfunction in bipolar disorder.
C. Less reduction in manic symptoms during treatment.
D. An increasing role for these hyperintensities in bipolar cognitive impairment with increasing age.
E. All of the above.

The correct response is option E.

The presence of hyperintensities may be especially important in late-life bipolar disorder because of their impact on treatment response and severity of illness. In bipolar studies, data are very limited, but MRI hyperintensities are associated with longer hospital stays (Dupont et al. 1990) and more frequent rehospitalizations (McDonald et al. 1999). In a small sample ($N=9$), Young (personal communication 2002) noted that the presence of periventricular hyperintensities is associated with less reduction in manic symptoms over 3 weeks in a naturalistic treatment setting. Also, hyperintensities appear to be related to cognitive changes. Bearden et al. (2001), reviewing the literature, concluded that hyperintensities play an increasing role in bipolar cognitive impairment with increasing age and chronicity of disorder, and that they may be considered a risk modifier for cognitive dysfunction in bipolar disorder. **(pp. 307–308)**

16.5 Which of the following atypical antipsychotic agents is approved by the U.S. Food and Drug Administration (FDA) for the treatment of acute depression?

A. Aripiprazole.
B. Olanzapine.
C. Ziprasidone.
D. Risperidone.
E. Quetiapine.

The correct response is option E.

Increasingly, the atypical antipsychotic agents are being used for the treatment of various phases of bipolar disorder. Five (olanzapine, risperidone, quetiapine, ziprasidone, aripiprazole) are currently approved by the FDA for the treatment of acute mania; two (olanzapine/fluoxetine, quetiapine) are FDA approved for the treatment of acute depression; and two (olanzapine, aripiprazole) are approved for the treatment of the maintenance phase. However, there are limited data for their efficacy in the geriatric-specific population. **(p. 311)**

References

Bearden CE, Hoffman KM, Cannon TD: The neuropsychology and neuroanatomy of bipolar affective disorder: a critical review. Bipolar Disord 3:106–150, 2001

Beyer J, Kuchibhatla M, Gersing K, et al: Medical comorbidity in an outpatient bipolar clinical population. Neuropsychopharmacology 30:401–404, 2005

Dupont RM, Jernigan TL, Butters N, et al: Subcortical abnormalities detected in bipolar affective disorder using magnetic resonance imaging: clinical and neuropsychological significance. Arch Gen Psychiatry 47:55–59, 1990

Goodwin FK, Jamison KR: Manic-Depressive Illness. New York, Oxford University Press, 1990

Hirschfeld RM, Lewis L, Vornik LA: Perceptions and impact of bipolar disorder: how far have we really come? Results of the national depressive and manic-depressive association 2000 survey of individuals with bipolar disorder. J Clin Psychiatry 64:161–174, 2003

Klap R, Unroe KT, Unutzer J: Caring for mental illness in the United States: a focus on older adults. Am J Geriatr Psychiatry 11:517–524, 2003

McDonald WM, Tupler LA, Marsteller FA, et al: Hyperintense lesions on magnetic resonance images in bipolar disorder. Biol Psychiatry 45:965–971, 1999

Unutzer J, Simon G, Pabiniak C, et al: The treated prevalence of bipolar disorder in a large staff-model HMO. Psychiatr Serv 49:1072–1078, 1998

Weissman MM, Leaf PJ, Tischler GL, et al: Affective disorders in five United States communities. Psychol Med 18:141–153, 1988

Chapter 17

Schizophrenia and Paranoid Disorders

Select the single best response for each question.

17.1 Recent data suggest that patients with late-onset schizophrenia, in comparison with early-onset patients, have a lower prevalence of

    A. The paranoid subtype.
    B. Persecutory delusions.
    C. Organized delusions.
    D. Auditory hallucinations.
    E. Negative symptoms.

The correct response is option E.

Data from the Sam and Rose Stein Institute for Research and Aging suggest a higher prevalence of the paranoid subtype of schizophrenia among patients with late-onset schizophrenia (approximately 75%) than among patients with early-onset schizophrenia (approximately 50%) (Jeste et al. 1997). Patients with late-onset schizophrenia tend to have more organized delusions, auditory hallucinations or hallucinations with a running commentary, and persecutory delusions with and without hallucinations (Howard et al. 2000). Patients with late-onset schizophrenia have lower levels of negative symptoms, on average, than patients with early-onset schizophrenia. **(p. 319)**

17.2 Factors distinguishing patients with very-late-onset schizophrenia-like psychosis (VLOSLP), wherein the onset of psychosis is after age 60 years, from "true" schizophrenia patients, include all of the following *except*

    A. Lower genetic load.
    B. Less evidence of early childhood maladjustment.
    C. Less risk of tardive dyskinesia.
    D. A relative lack of thought disorder.
    E. More evidence of a neurodegenerative process.

The correct response is option C.

Factors distinguishing patients with VLOSLP from "true" schizophrenia patients include a lower genetic load, less evidence of early childhood maladjustment, a relative lack of thought disorder and negative symptoms (including blunted affect), greater risk of tardive dyskinesia, and evidence of a neurodegenerative rather than a neurodevelopmental process (Andreasen 1999; Howard et al. 1997). Although the term was initially considered a catchall phrase for several different entities, recent research suggests that VLOSLP may be a distinct entity. It has been noted to be more common in immigrant populations, suggesting that psychosocial factors play a role (Mitter et al. 2005). **(p. 320)**

17.3 Which of the following is the most common symptom in psychosis of Alzheimer's disease?

    A. Visual hallucinations.
    B. Delusions.
    C. Depression.
    D. Disorganization of speech and behavior.
    E. Auditory hallucinations.

The correct response is option B.

Two common psychotic symptoms in Alzheimer's disease are misidentification of caregivers and delusions of theft (Jeste et al. 2007). Schneiderian first-rank symptoms, such as hearing multiple voices talking to one another or hearing a running commentary on the patient's actions, are rare (Burns et al. 1990a, 1990b). Disorganization of speech and behavior and negative symptoms are also uncommon (Jeste et al. 2007). **(pp. 321–322)**

17.4 In a consensus survey of 48 American experts on the treatment of older adults with late-life schizophrenia, the first-line medication treatment recommendation was

    A. Aripiprazole.
    B. Clozapine.
    C. Olanzapine.
    D. Quetiapine.
    E. Risperidone.

The correct response is option E.

Because of the dearth of randomized, controlled data, Alexopoulos et al. (2004) conducted a consensus survey of 48 American experts on the use of antipsychotic drugs in older adults. The experts' first-line recommendation for late-life schizophrenia was risperidone (1.25–3.5 mg/day). Second-line recommendations included quetiapine (100–300 mg/day), olanzapine (7.5–15 mg/day), and aripiprazole (15–30 mg/day). There was limited support for the use of clozapine, ziprasidone, and high-potency conventional antipsychotics. **(p. 324)**

17.5 Recently the U.S. Food and Drug Administration (FDA) issued a black-box warning for the use of atypical antipsychotics in elderly dementia patients. Which adverse event was noted to occur at a higher rate in this patient population?

    A. Hyperlipidemia.
    B. Diabetes.
    C. Hypertension.
    D. Stroke.
    E. Weight gain.

The correct response is option D.

The use of atypical antipsychotics in elderly patients with dementia has been associated with both cerebrovascular adverse events (CVAEs) and death, leading to black-box warnings by the FDA. Currently, risperidone, olanzapine, and aripiprazole carry black-box warnings for stroke risk in older patients with dementia. The data for quetiapine in this population are more limited than for risperidone, olanzapine, and aripiprazole. The attribution of risk of CVAEs to atypical antipsychotics is limited, however, in that these studies were not designed to determine a cause-and-effect relationship between atypical antipsychotics and CVAEs, and serious CVAEs were not operationally defined in the trials. **(pp. 325–326)**

17.6 In the National Institute of Mental Health Clinical Antipsychotic Trials of Intervention Effectiveness Alzheimer's disease (CATIE-AD) trial, which was the largest non-industry-sponsored trial of atypical antipsychotics for psychosis or agitation/aggression in people with dementia, which of the following agents was found to be better than placebo for the primary outcome measure?

A. Aripiprazole.
B. Olanzapine.
C. Quetiapine.
D. Risperidone.
E. No agent.

The correct response is option E.

In the CATIE-AD trial—the largest ($N = 421$) non-industry-sponsored trial of atypical antipsychotics for psychosis or agitation/aggression in people with dementia—olanzapine, quetiapine, and risperidone were no better than placebo for the primary outcome (time to discontinuation for any reason) (Schneider et al. 2006). Time to discontinuation due to lack of efficacy favored olanzapine and risperidone, whereas time to discontinuation due to adverse events favored placebo. **(p. 325)**

References

Alexopoulos GS, Streim J, Carpenter D, et al: Using antipsychotic agents in older patients. J Clin Psychiatry 65:5–99, 2004

Andreasen NC: I don't believe in late onset schizophrenia, in Late-Onset Schizophrenia. Edited by Howard R, Rabins PV, Castle DJ. Philadelphia, PA, Wrightson Biomedical, 1999, pp 111–123

Burns A, Jacoby R, Levy R: Psychiatric phenomena in Alzheimer's disease, I: disorders of thought content. Br J Psychiatry 157:72–76, 1990a

Burns A, Jacoby R, Levy R: Psychiatric phenomena in Alzheimer's disease, II: disorders of perception. Br J Psychiatry 157:76–81, 1990b

Howard R, Graham C, Sham P, et al: A controlled family study of late-onset non-affective psychosis (late paraphrenia). Br J Psychiatry 170:511–514, 1997

Howard R, Rabins PV, Seeman MV, et al: Late-onset schizophrenia and very-late-onset schizophrenia-like psychosis: an international consensus. Am J Psychiatry 157:172–178, 2000

Jeste DV, Symonds LL, Harris MJ, et al: Non-dementia non-praecox dementia praecox? Late-onset schizophrenia. Am J Geriatr Psychiatry 5:302–317, 1997

Mitter P, Reeves S, Romero-Rubiales F, et al: Migrant status, age, gender and social isolation in very late-onset schizophrenia-like psychosis. Int J Geriatr Psychiatry 20:1046–1051, 2005

Schneider LS, Tariot PN, Dagerman KS, et al: Effectiveness of atypical antipsychotic drugs in patients with Alzheimer's disease. N Engl J Med 355:1525–1538, 2006

Chapter 18

Anxiety Disorders

Select the single best response for each question.

18.1 All of the anxiety disorders are associated with some degree of avoidance and arousal. Based on these shared and distinct features, the anxiety disorders can be grouped into categories based on the nature of their phenomenology. Which of the following disorders is grouped into the fear category?

    A. Panic disorder.
    B. Acute stress disorder.
    C. Obsessive-compulsive disorder (OCD).
    D. Generalized anxiety disorder (GAD).
    E. Posttraumatic stress disorder (PTSD).

The correct response is option A.

The eight DSM-IV-TR (American Psychiatric Association 2000) anxiety disorders—GAD, panic disorder, specific phobia, social phobia, agoraphobia, OCD, PTSD, and acute stress disorder—can be divided into three main categories based on the nature of their phenomenology: worry/distress disorders (GAD, PTSD, and acute stress disorder), fear disorders (panic disorder and the phobias), and OCD (Watson 2005). **(p. 333)**

18.2 Several large epidemiological studies were published that included a large sample of elderly persons. Which of the following anxiety disorders is at least as common in late life as in younger adults?

    A. Obsessive-compulsive disorder.
    B. Generalized anxiety disorder.
    C. Panic disorder.
    D. Phobias (specific and social).
    E. Posttraumatic stress disorder.

The correct response is option B.

These studies, conducted using the National Comorbidity Study Replication as a mixed-age comparator, suggest that GAD is at least as common in late life as it is in younger adults, whereas other anxiety disorders (particularly OCD, and probably panic disorder) are rarer (Table 18–1). Because only one of these studies surveyed PTSD (National Mental Health and Well-Being Study), it is likely that anxiety prevalence rates are underestimated among the other investigations. **(pp. 334–335)**

18.3 The central feature of generalized anxiety disorder is

    A. Irritability.
    B. Fear.
    C. Worry.
    D. Arousal.
    E. Avoidance.

The correct response is option C.

TABLE 18–1. Prevalence estimates of late-life anxiety disorders from epidemiological studies

| | Epidemiological studies in the elderly | | | | | |
	LASA	ECA	AMSTEL	NMHWS	CCHS	NCS-R (adults)
N	3,107		4,051	1,792	12,792	9,282
Age range	55–85	65+	65–84	65+	55+	18+
Prevalence						
Any anxiety disorder	10.2%	5.5%	N/A	4.4%	N/A	18.1%
Generalized anxiety disorder	7.3%	1.9%	3.2%	2.4%	N/A	3.1%
Phobic disorder	3.1%	4.8%	N/A	0.6% (social)	1.3% (social) 0.6% (agoraphobia)	8.7%
Panic disorder	1.0%	0.1%	N/A	0.8%	0.8%	2.7%
Obsessive-compulsive disorder	0.6%	0.8%	N/A	0.1%	N/A	1.0%
Posttraumatic stress disorder	N/A	N/A	N/A	1.0%	N/A	3.5%

Note. AMSTEL=Amsterdam Study of the Elderly; CCHS=Canadian Community Health Survey; ECA=Epidemiologic Catchment Area; LASA=Longitudinal Aging Study Amsterdam; NCS-R=National Comorbidity Study Replication; NMHWS=National Mental Health and Well-being Study. N/A=not applicable.

The central feature of GAD is worry or anticipation of future negative events. Also known as "anxious apprehension," worry is thought to be a separate form of anxiety from fear or "anxious arousal" as seen in the fear disorders (e.g., panic disorder). Phenomenologically, they are quite different: worry may wax and wane but does not have the intense episodic nature of panic attacks (although worry can itself precipitate panic attacks). As such, GAD has evolved diagnostically to be first considered as a residual state of phobic/panic anxiety, then as a disorder in its own right, and now, in the looming DSM-V era, as a close relative to MDD. Worry in DSM-IV-TR-diagnosed GAD must be excessive, difficult to control, and cause distress. The actual content of worry in late-life GAD has been noted to be similar to that in older adults without GAD—that is, concerns about health or disability, family relationships, or finances (Diefenbach et al. 2001). **(p. 336)**

18.4 Which of the following has been reported to be the most common anxiety disorder in older African American patients?

    A. Generalized anxiety disorder.
    B. Panic disorder.
    C. Obsessive-compulsive disorder.
    D. Social phobia.
    E. Posttraumatic stress disorder.

The correct response is option E.

A recent epidemiological report in older African American patients found that PTSD was the most common anxiety disorder in this population, with the highest 12-month prevalence of any mental disorder (Ford et al. 2007). These findings may have reflected methodological differences from other studies or real differences from Caucasians in this age group. Overall, the research in late-life PTSD is far behind its overall impact in terms of prevalence and morbidity (van Zelst et al. 2003). **(p. 338)**

18.5 Which of the following cognitive functions is usually not impaired in older patients with generalized anxiety disorder and may be even improved?

    A. Short-term memory.
    B. Recall.
    C. Long-term memory.
    D. Executive functioning.
    E. Delayed memory.

The correct response is option D.

Some reports examining neuropsychological features in late-life GAD have drawn on literature that demonstrates a relationship between anxiety symptoms and cognitive decline in older adults (e.g., Wetherell et al. 2002). A preliminary study comparing GAD patients, major depressive disorder (MDD) patients, and healthy elderly found impaired short-term and delayed memory in GAD but not executive deficits as seen in MDD (Mantella et al. 2007). Another study of late-life GAD found that more severe worry was associated with better executive function, in a measure of inhibitory control (Price and Mohlman 2007). These results are consistent with another study in late-life GAD that found increased anxiety severity was associated with memory impairments (Caudle et al. 2007). Similar findings have been reported in late-life PTSD (Yehuda et al. 2007). **(p. 339)**

18.6 Depressed elderly patients with comorbid anxiety, in contrast to depressed elderly individuals without anxiety, usually have

    A. Lower risk of suicide.
    B. Reduced response rate to treatment.
    C. Shorter time to achieve a response to treatment.
    D. Fewer somatic symptoms.
    E. Less suicidal ideation.

The correct response is option B.

The combination of anxiety and depression in elderly persons is a severe and often treatment-resistant illness. Depressed elderly with comorbid anxiety have greater somatic symptoms, greater suicidal ideation (Jeste et al. 2006; Lenze et al. 2000), and a higher risk of suicide (Allgulander and Lavori 1993). Many studies have demonstrated a longer time to response in depression, and/or a reduced response rate, in association with anxiety symptoms (Alexopoulos et al. 2005; Andreescu et al. 2007; Dew et al. 1997; Lenze et al. 2003; Mulsant et al. 1996) or an anxiety disorder (Flint and Rifat 1997; Steffens et al. 2005). The reason for these findings is unclear; it may simply be that the combination of two disorders results in higher symptom levels, which reduces the chance of remitting to "normal" levels of symptoms. **(p. 340)**

References

Alexopoulos GS, Katz IR, Bruce ML, et al: Remission in depressed geriatric primary care patients: a report from the PROSPECT study. The PROSPECT Group. Am J Psychiatry 162:718–724, 2005

Allgulander C, Lavori PW: Causes of death among 936 elderly patients with "pure" anxiety neurosis in Stockholm County, Sweden, and in patients with depressive neurosis or both diagnoses. Compr Psychiatry 34:299–302, 1993

American Psychiatric Association: Diagnostic and Statistical Manual of Mental Disorders, 4th Edition, Text Revision. Washington, DC, American Psychiatric Association, 2000

Andreescu C, Lenze EJ, Dew MA, et al: Effect of comorbid anxiety on treatment response and relapse risk in late-life depression: controlled study. Br J Psychiatry 190:344–349, 2007

Caudle DD, Senior AC, Wetherell JL, et al: Cognitive errors, symptom severity, and response to cognitive behavior therapy in older adults with generalized anxiety disorder. Am J Geriatr Psychiatry 15:680–689, 2007

Dew MA, Reynolds CF 3rd, Houck PR, et al: Temporal profiles of the course of depression during treatment: predictors of pathways toward recovery in the elderly. Arch Gen Psychiatry 54:1016–1024, 1997

Diefenbach GJ, Stanley MA, Beck JG: Worry content reported by older adults with and without generalized anxiety disorder. Aging Ment Health 5:269–274, 2001

Flint AJ, Rifat SL: Two-year outcome of elderly patients with anxious depression. Psychiatry Res 66:23–31, 1997

Ford BC, Bullard KM, Taylor RJ, et al: Lifetime and 12-month prevalence of DSM–IV disorders among older African Americans: findings from the National Survey of American Life (NSAL). Am J Geriatr Psychiatry 15:652–659, 2007

Jeste ND, Hays JC, Steffens DC: Clinical correlates of anxious depression among elderly patients with depression. J Affect Disord 90:37–41, 2006

Lenze EJ, Mulsant BH, Shear MK, et al: Comorbid anxiety disorders in depressed elderly patients. Am J Psychiatry 15:722–728, 2000

Lenze EJ, Mulsant BH, Dew MA, et al: Good treatment outcomes in late-life depression with comorbid anxiety. J Affect Disord 77:247–254, 2003

Mantella RC, Butters MA, Dew MA, et al: Cognitive impairment in late-life generalized anxiety disorder. Am J Geriatr Psychiatry 15:673–679, 2007

Mulsant BH, Reynolds CF, Shear MK, et al: Comorbid anxiety disorders in late-life depression. Anxiety 2:242–247, 1996

Price RB, Mohlman J: Inhibitory control and symptom severity in late life generalized anxiety disorder. Behav Res Ther 45:2628–2639, 2007

Steffens DC, McQuoid DR: Impact of symptoms of generalized anxiety disorder on the course of late-life depression. Am J Geriatr Psychiatry 13:40–47, 2005

van Zelst WH, de Beurs E, Beekman AT, et al: Prevalence and risk factors of posttraumatic stress disorder in older adults. Psychother Psychosom 72:333–342, 2003

Watson D: Rethinking the mood and anxiety disorders: a quantitative hierarchical model for DSM-V. J Abnorm Psychol 114:522–536, 2005

Wetherell JL, Reynolds CA, Gatz M, et al: Anxiety, cognitive performance, and cognitive decline in normal aging. J Gerontol Psychol Sci 57B:P246–P255, 2002

Yehuda R, Golier JA, Tischler L, et al: Hippocampal volume in aging combat veterans with and without posttraumatic stress disorder: relation to risk and resilience factors. J Psychiatr Res 41:435–445, 2007

Chapter 19

Somatoform Disorders

Select the single best response for each question.

19.1 The diagnostic feature of somatization disorder that is most difficult to establish in elderly patients is

A. Pain at four or more sites.
B. Physical complaints not fully explained by the medical workup.
C. Onset prior to age 30.
D. Relevant physical findings.
E. Comorbid illness.

The correct response is option C.

The most difficult diagnostic feature to establish in elderly patients is the onset of symptoms before age 30, because such history can rarely be accurately determined. In addition, the presence of multiple physical symptoms in excess of what would be expected is a relative factor in late life, given the high incidence of comorbid illnesses. Somatization disorder tends to run a chronic course, with the majority of individuals demonstrating consistent symptom patterns as they age, even into later life (Pribor et al. 1994). **(p. 348)**

19.2 Undifferentiated somatoform disorder is defined by all of the following *except*

A. Presence of one or more physical complaints.
B. Symptoms last at least 6 months.
C. Symptoms cannot be fully explained by appropriate medical workup.
D. Symptoms result in considerable impairment.
E. Symptoms include pain at four or more sites.

The correct response is option E.

Undifferentiated somatoform disorder is defined by the presence of one or more physical complaints, lasting at least 6 months, that cannot be fully explained by appropriate medical workup and that result in considerable social, occupational, or functional impairment. **(p. 348)**

19.3 Which of the following is *not* a risk factor for conversion disorder?

A. Being male.
B. Physical abuse.
C. Personality disorder.
D. Other neurological illnesses.
E. Sexual abuse.

The correct response is option A.

Risk factors for conversion disorder include physical and sexual abuse, personality disorder, and other neurological illnesses (O'Sullivan et al. 2007; Roelofs et al. 2002; Sar et al. 2004). Conversion disorder in late life may be even more likely to be associated with an actual comorbid neurological disorder. The prognosis is variable and depends on several factors including the degree of functional impairment and psychiatric comorbidity, and the type of symptoms. (p. 349)

19.4   What is the most common medical complaint in elderly persons?

    A. Dizziness.
    B. Pain.
    C. Constipation.
    D. Insomnia.
    E. Gait instability.

The correct response is option B.

Pain is the most common medical complaint in elderly persons, with pain caused by musculoskeletal disease (e.g., osteoarthritis, back pain, headache) being the most common type of pain (Leveille et al. 2001). Nearly 50% of elderly individuals have chronic pain, and the percentage approaches 70% for those in long-term care (Otis and McGeeney 2000). Persistent pain is associated with significant functional and social impairment (Scudds and Ostbye 2001) as well as comorbid psychiatric symptoms, including depression, insomnia, and substance abuse. (pp. 349–350)

19.5   A number of factors have been associated with an increased risk for somatoform disorders. Which of the following is one of these factors?

    A. Male gender.
    B. Serious illness late in life.
    C. Higher educational level.
    D. Childhood abuse.
    E. High socioeconomic status.

The correct response is option D.

The causes of somatoform disorders are usually multifactorial and are often rooted in early developmental experiences and personality traits. For example, somatization and all somatoform disorders have been associated with the experience of serious illness early in life (Stuart and Noyes 1999), childhood abuse (Roelofs et al. 2002; Samelius et al. 2007; Waldinger et al. 2006), dissociative amnesia (Brown et al. 2005), significant psychological stress (Hollifield et al. 1999; Ritsner et al. 2000), and the personality traits of alexithymia and neuroticism (Bailey and Henry 2007; De Gucht 2003; Phillips and McElroy 2000). As noted throughout the chapter, somatoform disorders are also highly associated with comorbid depression, anxiety and panic disorders, substance abuse, and personality disorders (Noyes et al. 2001; Sar et al. 2004). (p. 351)

References

Bailey PE, Henry JD: Alexithymia, somatization and negative affect in a community sample. Psychiatry Res 150:13–20, 2007

Brown RJ, Schrag A, Trimble MR: Dissociation, childhood interpersonal trauma, and family functioning in patients with somatization disorder. Am J Psychiatry 162:899–905, 2005

De Gucht V: Stability of neuroticism and alexithymia in somatization. Compr Psychiatry 44:466–471, 2003

Hollifield M, Tuttle L, Paine S, et al: Hypochondriasis and somatization related to personality and attitudes towards self. Psychosomatics 40:387–395, 1999

Leveille SG, Ling S, Hochberg MC, et al: Widespread musculoskeletal pain and the progression of disability in older disabled women. Ann Intern Med 135:1038–1046, 2001

Noyes R Jr, Langbehn DR, Happel RL, et al: Personality dysfunction among somatizing patients. Psychosomatics 42:320–329, 2001

O'Sullivan SS, Spillane JE, McMahon EM: Clinical characteristics and outcome of patients diagnosed with psychogenic nonepileptic seizures: a 5-year review. Epilepsy Behav 11:77–84, 2007

Otis JAD, McGeeney B: Managing pain in the elderly. Clin Geriatr 8:48–62, 2000

Phillips KA, McElroy SL: Personality disorders and traits in patients with body dysmorphic disorder. Compr Psychiatry 41:229–236, 2000

Pribor EF, Smith DS, Yutzy SH: Somatization disorder in elderly patients. J Geriatr Psychiatry 2:109–117, 1994

Ritsner M, Ponizovsky A, Kurs R, et al: Somatization in an immigrant population in Israel: a community survey of prevalence, risk factors, and help-seeking behavior. Am J Psychiatry 157:385–392, 2000

Roelofs K, Keijsers GP, Hoogduin KA, et al: Childhood abuse in patients with conversion disorder. Am J Psychiatry 159:1908–1913, 2002

Samelius L, Wijma B, Wingren G, et al: Somatization in abused women. J Womens Health 6:909–918, 2007

Sar V, Akyüz G, Kundakçi T: Childhood trauma, dissociation, and psychiatric comorbidity in patients with conversion disorder. Am J Psychiatry 161:2271–2276, 2004

Scudds RJ, Ostbye T: Pain and pain-related interference with function in older Canadians: the Canadian Study of Health and Aging. Disabil Rehabil 23:654–664, 2001

Stuart S, Noyes R Jr: Attachment and interpersonal communication in somatization. Psychosomatics 40:34–43, 1999

Waldinger RJ, Schulz MS, Barsky AJ, et al: Mapping the road from childhood trauma to adult somatization: the role of attachment. Psychosom Med 68:129–135, 2006

Chapter 20

Sexual Disorders

Select the single best response for each question.

20.1 Which of the following is the first stage of the normal sexual response cycle?

A. Plateau.
B. Arousal.
C. Orgasm.
D. Desire.
E. Resolution.

The correct response is option D.

The first stage of the five-stage model, *desire*, involves physical and psychological urges to seek out and respond to sexual interaction. This drive is centered in the limbic system of the brain, particularly in the hypothalamus, and is stimulated in both sexes by testosterone. Desire is intimately linked to the physiological process of sexual *excitement* or *arousal* (the second stage); it is difficult for one to exist without the other. In both men and women, sexual arousal can be triggered by thoughts and fantasies or by direct physical stimulation. Autonomic nervous stimulation leads to predictable physiological responses, including increased muscle tone, increases in heart and respiratory rates, and increased blood flow to the genitals (vasocongestion). In men, these responses result in penile erection, whereas in women, they result in vaginal lubrication and swelling of breast and genital tissues, especially the clitoris. The relatively brief *plateau* stage is characterized by a sense of impending *orgasm* and is followed by orgasm and then a refractory period of relaxation called *resolution*. **(p. 359)**

20.2 In women, the most significant changes in the sexual response cycle occur during menopause. Which of the following changes is caused by a decrease in testosterone?

A. Atrophy of urogenital tissue.
B. Less intense orgasms.
C. Decreased libido.
D. Decrease in vaginal size.
E. Reduced vaginal lubrication.

The correct response is option C.

Normal aging produces several changes in the sexual response cycle (see Table 20–1). In women, the most significant changes occur during menopause, a 2- to 10-year period that usually ends in the early 50s. The decline and eventual cessation of ovarian estrogen production during menopause leads to important changes in sexual function, including atrophy of urogenital tissue, a decrease in vaginal size, and diminished vaginal lubrication, vasocongestion, and erotic sensitivity of nipple, clitoral, and vulvar tissue. As a result, sexual desire may decrease, sexual arousal may require more time, sexual intercourse may be more uncomfortable because of reduced lubrication of vaginal and clitoral tissue, and orgasms may be felt as less intense. Up to 85% of menopausal women also experience symptoms such as hot flashes, head and neck aches, mood changes, and excess fatigue. During menopause, women also experience decreases in testosterone production that may lead to diminished libido (Nappi et al. 2006). **(pp. 359–360)**

TABLE 20–1. Normal age-related changes in sexual function

Men

Testosterone production modestly decreases, with unpredictable effect on sexual function.

Sperm count changes minimally, but amount of functional sperm and rate of conception decrease.

There are no predictable changes in sexual desire (libido).

Increased tactile stimulation is needed for sexual arousal.

Erections take longer to achieve and are more difficult to sustain.

Penile rigidity decreases because of decreases in blood flow and smooth muscle relaxation.

Sensation of urgency during plateau stage is diminished.

Ejaculation is less forceful, with decreased ejaculate volume.

Refractory period increases by hours to days.

Women

During menopause, estrogen production decreases and eventually stops.

Sexual desire (libido) may decrease due in part to decreased testosterone levels.

Blood supply to pelvic region is reduced.

Vagina shortens and narrows. Vaginal mucosa is thinner and less lubricated.

During arousal, vaginal lubrication and swelling occur more slowly and are decreased.

Sexual arousal may take longer and may require increased stimulation.

During orgasm, strength and amount of vaginal contractions decrease.

Source.   Goodwin and Agronin 1997; Metz and Miner 1995; Spector et al. 1996.

20.3   As men age, which of the following sexual parameters increases instead of decreases?

    A. Volume of ejaculate.

    B. Refractory period.

    C. Libido.

    D. Bone and muscle mass.

    E. Frequency of erections.

The correct response is option B.

Compared with women, the sexual changes in aging men occur more gradually with a less predictable time frame (Metz and Miner 1995; Westheimer and Lopater 2002). As men age, desire may involve less anticipatory physical arousal, and sexual arousal and orgasm may take longer to achieve. Older men require more physical stimulation to achieve erections, which tend to be less frequent, less durable, and less reliable. The volume of ejaculate during orgasm is decreased. In older men, the resolution or refractory stage is much longer, lasting hours to days instead of minutes to hours as in younger men. Testosterone levels in men decline 35% on average by age 80, although some men have more significant declines, with levels dropping below 200 ng/dL, termed *hypogonadism* (Morley 2003). Some researchers have suggested the existence of a male menopause or *andropause* resulting from declining testosterone levels and involving a symptom complex that includes decreased libido and sexual function; diminished bone and muscle mass, muscle power, and body hair; and decreased lean body mass (Heaton and Morales 2001; Morley and Perry 2003; Westheimer and Lopater 2002). **(p. 360)**

20.4   In older men, especially those over the age of 70, the most common sexual disorder is

    A. Hypoactive sexual desire.

    B. Inhibited orgasm.

    C. Premature ejaculation.

    D. Sexual aversion.

    E. Erectile dysfunction.

The correct response is option E.

Erectile dysfunction is the most common form of sexual dysfunction in older men, affecting more than 50% of men ages 40–70 years and nearly 70% of men age 70 years or older (Althof and Seftel 1995; Feldman et al. 1994). **(p. 361)**

20.5 You diagnose major depression in a 70-year-old man. He wants you to prescribe an antidepressant with the fewest sexual side effects. He is on no other medications and has no significant medical illnesses. Which of the following antidepressants do you recommend because it has the lowest rate of reported sexual dysfunction?

    A. Bupropion.
    B. Venlafaxine.
    C. Imipramine.
    D. Sertraline.
    E. Mirtazapine.

The correct response is option A.

Erectile dysfunction, delayed or inhibited orgasm, and/or a decrease in desire is experienced by 10%–60% of men taking selective serotonin reuptake inhibitors, venlafaxine, or tricyclic antidepressants (Montejo et al. 2001; Segraves 1998). Lower rates of sexual dysfunction have been associated with the antidepressants mirtazapine (25%), bupropion (5%–15%), and nefazodone (8%) (Kavoussi et al. 1997; Montejo et al. 2001). **(p. 363)**

20.6 You prescribe an antidepressant for a 70-year-old man with major depression and no comorbid medical conditions. He calls you 2 weeks after starting the medication and states that his mood has improved greatly; however, he is experiencing some sexual side effects. What would be the most logical first step in addressing his sexual complaints?

    A. Encourage him to stop the medication over the weekend and encourage him to attempt sexual intercourse.
    B. Stop the medication and replace it with another antidepressant.
    C. Reduce the dose of the medication.
    D. Continue the medication and wait to see if the side effects decrease.
    E. Prescribe an antidote, such as sildenafil.

The correct response is option D.

When medication side effects impair sexual function, physicians can consider several options (Goodwin and Agronin 1997; Labbate et al. 2003; Zajecka 2001). The first step is to continue administering the medication and wait for tolerance to develop; many side effects diminish or disappear after several weeks. If no change occurs, dose reduction can be tried. For certain medications, such as antidepressants with short half-lives, a drug holiday in which administration of the medication is temporarily stopped for a day or two (such as for a weekend) can result in transient improvement in sexual function (Rothschild 1995). However, there is a risk of recurrence of psychiatric symptoms during this holiday. Ultimately, the clinician may have to consider replacing the medication with an agent that has less potential for sexual side effects, such as bupropion or mirtazapine (Gelenberg et al. 2000). **(pp. 364–365)**

20.7 Hypoactive sexual desire in older women is caused by a number of psychological and physical factors. Which of the following is **not** one of these factors?

    A. Poor self-image.
    B. Increased estrogen production.
    C. Decreased free testosterone.
    D. Negative societal attitudes of sexuality in late life.
    E. Internalized negative images of sexuality in older persons.

The correct response is option B.

Hypoactive sexual desire is a significant sexual problem for women across the life span and involves multiple psychological and physical factors. In some older women, loss of libido results from a poor self-image—brought about by age-associated losses of physical strength and beauty—and from changes in sexual function caused by cessation of estrogen production during menopause. An older woman's ability to see herself as a sexual being can be further eroded by exposure to negative societal attitudes and negative images of sexuality in late life. Unfortunately, many women internalize these distorted, ageist beliefs. Treatment of low desire must begin with sex education and counseling to counter those psychological barriers. Estrogen replacement therapy may help improve sexual arousal and comfort, which in turn may lead to increased desire.

The critical physiological cause of low desire in women, however, appears to be the menopause-associated reduction in levels of free testosterone. Testosterone replacement therapy has been beneficial in women with hypoactive sexual desire (Basson 1999; Buster et al. 2005; Shifren et al. 2006), although side effects can include weight gain, virilization (e.g., growth of facial and chest hair, lowering of the voice), suppression of clotting factors, and even liver damage (Kingsberg et al. 2007). Sildenafil therapy has also been studied in women with sexual dysfunction (hypoactive desire, orgasmic disorder, or dyspareunia) associated with female sexual arousal disorder, but though well tolerated, it did not lead to improvement (Basson et al. 2002). **(pp. 367–368)**

References

Althof SE, Seftel AD: The evaluation and management of erectile dysfunction. Psychiatr Clin North Am 18:171–192, 1995

Basson R: Androgen replacement for women. Can Fam Physician 45:2100–2107, 1999

Basson R, McInnes R, Smith MD, et al: Efficacy and safety of sildenafil in estrogenized women with sexual dysfunction associated with female sexual arousal disorder. J Womens Health Gend Based Med 1:367-377, 2002

Buster JE, Kingsberg SA, Aguirre O, et al: Testosterone patch for low sexual desire in surgically menopausal women: a randomized trial. Obstet Gynecol 105 (5 part 1):944–952, 2005

Feldman HA, Goldstein I, Hatzichristou DG, et al: Impotence and its medical and psychosocial correlates: results of the Massachusetts Male Aging Study. J Urol 151:54–61, 1994

Gelenberg AJ, McGahuey C, Laukes C, et al: Mirtazapine substitution in SSRI-induced sexual dysfunction. J Clin Psychiatry 61:356–360, 2000

Goodwin AJ, Agronin ME: A Women's Guide to Overcoming Sexual Fear and Pain. Oakland, CA, New Harbinger, 1997

Heaton JP, Morales A: Andropause—a multisystem disease. Can J Urol 8:1213–1222, 2001

Kavoussi RJ, Segraves RT, Hughes AR, et al: Double-blind comparison of bupropion sustained release and sertraline in depressed outpatients. J Clin Psychiatry 58:532–537, 1997

Kingsberg S, Shifren J, Wekselman K, et al: Evaluation of the clinical relevance of benefits associated with transdermal testosterone treatment in postmenopausal women with hypoactive sexual desire disorder. J Sex Med 4 (part 1): 1001–1008, 2007

Labbate LA, Croft HA, Oleshansky MA: Antidepressant-related erectile dysfunction: management via avoidance, switching antidepressants, antidotes, and adaptation. J Clin Psychiatry 64 (suppl 10):11–19, 2003

Metz ME, Miner MH: Male "menopause," aging, and sexual function: a review. Sex Disabil 13:287–307, 1995

Montejo AL, Llorca G, Izquierdo JA: Incidence of sexual dysfunction associated with antidepressant agents: a prospective multicenter study of 1022 outpatients. Spanish Working Group for the Study of Psychotropic-Related Sexual Dysfunction. J Clin Psychiatry 62 (suppl 3):10–21, 2001

Morley JE: Testosterone and behavior. Clin Geriatric Med 19:605–616, 2003

Morley JE, Perry HM 3rd: Andropause: an old concept in new clothing. Clin Geriatric Med 19:507–528, 2003

Nappi RE, Wawra K, Schmitt S: Hypoactive sexual desire disorder in postmenopausal women. Gynecol Endocrinol 22:318–323, 2006

Rothschild AJ: Selective serotonin reuptake inhibitor–induced sexual dysfunction: efficacy of a drug holiday. Am J Psychiatry 152:1514–1516, 1995

Segraves RT: Antidepressant-induced sexual dysfunction. J Clin Psychiatry 59 (suppl 4):48–54, 1998

Shifren JL, Davis SR, Moreau M, et al: Testosterone patch for the treatment of hypoactive sexual desire disorder in naturally menopausal women: results from the INTIMATE NM1 Study. Menopause 13:770–779, 2006

Spector IP, Rosen RC, Leiblum SR: Sexuality, in Psychiatric Care in the Nursing Home. Edited by Reichman WE, Katz PR. New York, Oxford University Press, 1996, pp 133–150

Westheimer RK, Lopater S: Human Sexuality: A Psychosocial Perspective. Philadelphia, PA, Lippincott Williams & Wilkins, 2002

Zajecka J: Strategies for the treatment of antidepressant-related sexual dysfunction: management via avoidance, switching antidepressants, antidotes, and adaptation. J Clin Psychiatry 64 (suppl 10):11–19, 2001

Chapter 21

Bereavement

Select the single best response for each question.

21.1 Numerous theoretical perspectives on the function and process of bereavement have been developed over the years. Who believed that any involuntary separation, including bereavement, gives rise to many forms of attachment behavior that reflect the person's desire to reunite with the lost person?

    A. Bierhals.
    B. Bowlby.
    C. Freud.
    D. Lindemann.
    E. Rosenblatt.

The correct response is option B.

Bowlby (1961) posited that any involuntary separation, including bereavement, gives rise to many forms of attachment behavior (such as separation anxiety and pining) that reflect the person's desire to reunite with the lost person. Thus, the function of bereavement is not a surrendering of attachment but rather an attempt to regain a sense of connection with the lost object of attachment. With time, these behaviors were thought to dissipate through a series of stages, including shock, protest, despair, and, finally, breakage of the bond and adjustment to a new self.

Early work on adjustment to permanent losses emphasized that mourning was a process whereby the bereaved gradually "surrendered" their attachment to the lost loved one by engaging in certain specific psychological and behavioral tasks that occurred at appropriate time points during the bereavement (Freud 1917[1915]/1957; Lindemann 1944). This process was thought to be necessary for the individual to develop new constructive attachments to other people entering his or her life.

Although stage theories of adaptation have been widely accepted by health care professionals, little empirical evidence exists to support these theories. For example, although stage theories would predict an eventual end stage where grieving ceases, grief symptoms often do not abate in elderly widows and widowers (see, for example, Bierhals et al. 1995).

Bereavement, as Rosenblatt (1996) contended, is a dynamic process that may continue for a number of years and even for the remainder of one's life. Also, bereaved individuals do not proceed from one clearly identifiable phase to another in an orderly fashion, a fact particularly true of older adults. **(p. 376)**

21.2 Several psychiatrists have proposed models of bereavement that involve phases or stages of reaction to the death of a loved one. Usually three stages are described. Which of the following is characteristic of the second or middle stage?

    A. Emotional numbness.
    B. Identity reconstruction.
    C. Cognitive confusion.
    D. Yearning and protest.
    E. Shock and disbelief.

The correct response is option D.

The second phase generally begins as the numbness and anxiety start to decrease. During this period, family and friends gradually become less available and often convey the message that the bereaved one should be getting on with life and should be getting over the grief, although the individual is far from ready to do so. The second phase is described as a time of "yearning and protest," during which the bereaved may actively search for the deceased (Parkes 1972). They may seek out things that remind them of their loved one or go to places often frequented by the deceased. They may also have a strong sense of the presence of their lost loved one, such as seeing someone that reminds them of the deceased and for a moment feeling certain that it must be them. Vivid experiences of auditory and visual hallucinations of the deceased often occur as a normal part of grieving. Although these experiences may be startling at first glance, they often are reported as positive or comforting (Grimby 1993; Rees 1971).

Parkes's (1972) first phase begins at the time of the death and persists for several weeks. Shock and disbelief, combined with emotional numbness and cognitive confusion, characterize this period, and intense free-floating anxiety and sharp mood fluctuations occur as well. Specific somatic symptoms include sleeplessness, loss of appetite, and vague muscular aches and pains, and these symptoms lead to increased contact with primary care physicians and, commonly, requests for medication.

The final phase is often referred to as "identity reconstruction" (Lopata 1996). During this period the bereaved person gradually reinvests the psychic energy that has been completely focused on the lost loved one into new relationships and activities. **(pp. 376–377)**

21.3 Bonnano et al. collected data on 205 older adults several years prior to the death of their spouse and again at 6 and 18 months postloss. Five patterns of adjustment were identified based on pre- and postloss levels of adjustment. All of the following are among these patterns *except*

    A. Chronic grief.
    B. Resilience.
    C. Normal grief.
    D. Chronic depression.
    E. Denial.

The correct response is option E.

A study by Bonnano et al. (2002) examined patterns of depression and recovery following loss based on data collected as a part of the Changing Lives of Older Couples study. Prospective data reflecting level of depression, grief, and psychosocial functioning were obtained from 205 older adults several years prior to the death of their spouse and again at 6 and 18 months postloss. Five patterns of adjustment were identified, based on pre- and postloss levels of adjustment. Those patterns include chronic grief (good adjustment preloss followed by chronic poor adjustment), chronic depression (poor adjustment at all three time points), depression followed by improvement (poor adjustment preloss, with improvement at either 6 or 18 months), common/normal grief (good preloss functioning with a decline at 6 months and subsequent improvement at 18 months) and resilience (good adjustment at all three time points). **(pp. 381–382)**

21.4 A number of studies have been undertaken to identify elders at risk for negative outcomes after spousal loss. Which of the following variables is generally *not* associated with prolonged or complicated bereavement?

    A. Death by suicide.
    B. Intense negative emotions at 2 months postloss.
    C. Making sense of the loss.
    D. Unexpected death.
    E. Being a widower.

The correct response is option C.

Bereaved individuals who report that they are able to make sense of a loss report better adjustment in the first year after the loss, while the ability to see the benefit in a loss (e.g., through making the bereaved person stronger or through greater valuing of friends and family) is associated with better adjustment later in the bereavement process (Davis et al. 1998).

Stroebe et al. (2001) concluded that "widowers are indeed at relatively higher risk [of death] than widows, and, given that death is the most extreme consequence of bereavement, much weight may be attached to this finding."

Violent, stigmatized (as in the case of AIDS), or unexpected deaths generally are associated with poorer adaptation (O'Neil 1989; Osterweis et al. 1984; Parkes and Weiss 1983). Farberow et al. (1987) compared older adults whose spouses had died of natural causes with older adults whose spouses had committed suicide and found that the effect of the suicide on the survivor was not notably different than the effects of other modes of death during the early period of bereavement. However, the expected decline in level of depression and other symptoms by the end of 1 year did not occur in those grieving the loss of a loved one by suicide.

Burton et al. (2006) found an association between unexpected death and depression in older adults both 6 and 18 months postloss. Further research is necessary to determine the long-term course of symptoms following the violent or unexpected death of a loved one.

Lund et al. (1993) found that intense negative emotions at 2 months postloss—such as a desire to die and frequent crying—were associated with poor coping 2 years later. **(pp. 382–384)**

21.5   Of the following preloss variables in spouses, which one has **not** consistently been found to be a risk factor for complicated bereavement?

   A. More negative ratings of preloss relationship satisfaction.
   B. Preloss depression.
   C. Poor self-esteem.
   D. Inadequate coping skills.
   E. Lack of social support.

The correct response is option A.

Though often discussed, the effects of preloss relationship satisfaction as a risk factor remain unclear (e.g., Parkes and Weiss 1983). Thus, relationship satisfaction may interact with several other variables, including general psychological health and a change in perspective on the relationship over the course of the bereavement process. Clearly, more research is needed in this area.

In work investigating the relationship between depression and later bereavement outcome (Gilewski et al. 1991), individuals with self-reported depression in the moderate to severe range were found to be at greatest risk for all other psychopathological symptoms, such as increased anxiety, hostility, interpersonal sensitivity, and other indices of global psychiatric distress. This result occurred whether their spouses had committed suicide or died of natural causes.

Several articles have suggested that bereaved elderly individuals with poor self-esteem and/or inadequate coping skills are at a greater risk for difficult bereavement. Johnson et al. (1986) conducted one of the few studies that directly addressed these variables in elders. As expected, individuals who early in bereavement reported themselves to be high in self-esteem and to be effective copers maintained a high self-esteem and remained effective copers throughout the first year of bereavement, whereas those who initially reported high stress levels generally had high levels of stress at subsequent times of measurement.

The role of social support is less ambiguous, overall. Since the publication of Cobb's (1976) seminal paper on the stress-buffering effects of this element, social support has been widely recognized as a moderator of many kinds of life stress. In a comprehensive review of the role of social support in mitigating the effects of bereavement, Stylianos and Vachon (1993) made the point that social support should be viewed as a multidimensional process, including such aspects as the size, structure, and quality of the network; types of support provided (and by whom); and the appraisal of the support. **(pp. 384–385)**

21.6 A number of psychological treatments for complicated bereavement have been studied. One such treatment is a 12-session phase-oriented strategy designed to help individuals work through emotional reactions to traumatic events. Which of the following is this treatment?

    A. Guided mourning.
    B. Cognitive-behavioral therapy.
    C. Time-limited psychodynamic psychotherapy.
    D. Interpersonal psychotherapy.
    E. Imaginal exposure.

The correct response is option C.

One of the more common psychodynamic therapies used with complicated bereavement is Horowitz's (1976) time-limited psychodynamic therapy. This 12-session phase-oriented strategy is designed to help individuals work through emotional reactions to traumatic life events. Careful attention is also paid to tailoring treatment to the patient's particular personality type.

Guided mourning is a brief, intensive, structured behavioral program that is helpful in the resolution of chronic grief (Mawson et al. 1981). The effectiveness of this approach has been replicated by Sireling et al. (1988). Ninety-minute sessions are held three times weekly for 2 weeks, with subsequent less intense follow-up for 28 weeks. The treatment is designed to help bereaved individuals repeatedly confront aspects of their loss in order to eventually diminish their negative effects through habituation.

Cognitive and cognitive-behavioral therapies of various forms have been used to treat patients with complex bereavement reactions. One such strategy focuses on core constructs known to be disrupted during intense grief (Viney 1990). As these are identified through self-monitoring and Socratic questioning during treatment sessions, the client learns methods of reconstructing shattered beliefs about the self and the present surroundings and future events.

A combination of medication and psychotherapy appears to be more effective than either alone when attempting to reduce psychiatric symptoms that occur with bereavement. For example, the late-life depression research group at the Western Psychiatric Institute in Pittsburgh, Pennsylvania, tested the efficacy of nortriptyline therapy, interpersonal psychotherapy, and combined treatment in elderly patients with bereavement-related major depression and reported that combined treatment was superior to either intervention alone, particularly among patients age 70 or older (Miller et al. 1997; Reynolds et al. 1999).

Researchers at the Western Psychiatric Institute (Frank et al. 1997; Shear et al. 2001, 2005) developed a treatment for complicated grief that involves principles similar to those featured in the treatment of posttraumatic stress disorder. The treatment for complicated grief includes a series of cognitive-behavioral techniques such as imaginal exposure to the death scene; in vivo, graded exposure to avoided death-related circumstances; mindful breathing; reminiscence of positive and negative memories of the loved one; and writing goodbye letters to the deceased person. Also integral to the treatment are homework assignments involving listening to tapes of imaginal exposure. Following the dual-process model, the treatment also involved motivational enhancement and goal setting to facilitate restorative goals. **(pp. 386–387)**

References

Bierhals AJ, Prigerson HG, Fasiczka A, et al: Gender differences in complicated grief among the elderly. Omega (Westport) 32:303–317, 1995

Bonanno GA, Wortman CB, Lehman DR, et al: Resilience to loss and chronic grief: a prospective study from pre-loss to 18 months post-loss. J Pers Soc Psychol 83:1150–1164, 2002

Bowlby J: Processes of mourning. Int J Psychoanal 42:317–340, 1961

Burton AM, Haley WE, Small BJ: Bereavement after caregiving or unexpected death: effects on elderly spouses. Aging Ment Health 10:319–326, 2006

Cobb S: Presidential Address-1976. Social support as a moderator of life stress. Psychosom Med 3:300–314, 1976

Davis CG, Nolen-Hoeksema S, Larson J: Making sense of loss and benefiting from the experience. J Pers Soc Psychol 75:561–574, 1998

Farberow NL, Gallagher DE, Gilewski MJ, et al: An examination of the early impact of bereavement on psychological distress in survivors of suicide. Gerontologist 27:592–598, 1987

Frank E, Prigerson HG, Shear MK, et al: Phenomenology and treatment of bereavement related distress in the elderly. Int Clin Psychopharmacol 12 (suppl):S25–S29, 1997

Freud S: Mourning and melancholia (1917[1915]), in The Standard Edition of the Complete Psychological Works of Sigmund Freud, Vol 14. Translated and edited by Strachey J. London, Hogarth, 1957, pp 237–260

Gilewski MJ, Farberow NL, Gallagher DE, et al: Interaction of depression and bereavement on mental health in the elderly. Psychol Aging 6:67–75, 1991

Grimby A: Bereavement among elderly people: grief reactions, post-bereavement hallucinations, and quality of life. Acta Psychiatr Scand 87:72–80, 1993

Horowitz MJ: Stress Response Syndromes. New York, Jason Aronson, 1976

Johnson RJ, Lund DA, Dimond M: Stress, self-esteem, and coping during bereavement among the elderly. Soc Psychol Q 49:273–279, 1986

Lindemann E: Symptomatology and management of acute grief. Am J Psychiatry 101:141–148, 1944

Lopata HZ: Current Widowhood: Myths and Realities. Thousand Oaks, CA, Sage, 1996

Lund DA, Caserta M, Dimond M: The course of spousal bereavement in later life, in Handbook of Bereavement. Edited by Stroebe MS, Stroebe W, Hansson R. Cambridge, United Kingdom, Cambridge University Press, 1993, pp 240–254

Mawson D, Marks IM, Ramm L, et al: Guided mourning for morbid grief: a controlled study. Br J Psychiatry 138:185–193, 1981

Miller MD, Wolfson L, Frank E, et al: Using interpersonal psychotherapy (IPT) in a combined psychotherapy/ medication research protocol with depressed elders: a descriptive report with case vignettes. J Psychother Pract Res 7:47–55, 1997

O'Neil M: Grief and bereavement in AIDS and aging. Generations 13:80–82, 1989

Osterweis M, Solomon F, Green M (eds): Bereavement: Reactions, Consequences, and Care. Washington, DC, National Academy Press, 1984

Parkes CM: Bereavement: Studies of Grief in Adult Life. New York, International Universities Press, 1972

Parkes CM, Weiss RS: Recovery From Bereavement. New York, Basic Books, 1983

Rees WD: The hallucinations of widowhood. Br Med J 4:37–41, 1971

Reynolds CF 3rd, Miller MD, Pasternak RE, et al: Treatment of bereavement-related major depressive episodes in later life: a controlled study of acute and continuation treatment with nortriptyline and interpersonal psychotherapy. Am J Psychiatry 156:202–208, 1999

Rosenblatt PC: Grief that does not end, in Continuing Bonds: New Understandings of Grief (Series in Death Education, Aging, and Health Care, 0275–3510). Edited by Klass D, Silverman PR, Nickman SL. Washington, DC, Taylor and Francis, 1996, pp 45–58

Shear MK, Frank E, Foa E, et al: Traumatic grief treatment: a pilot study. Am J Psychiatry 158:1506–1508, 2001

Shear [M]K, Frank E, Houck PR, et al: Treatment of complicated grief: a randomized controlled trial. JAMA 293:2601–2608, 2005

Sireling L, Cohen D, Marks I: Guided mourning for morbid grief: a controlled replication. Behav Ther 19:121–132, 1988

Stroebe MS, Stroebe W, Schut H: Gender differences in adjustment to bereavement: an empirical and theoretical review. Rev Gen Psychol 5:62–83, 2001

Stylianos S, Vachon M: The role of social support in bereavement, in Handbook of Bereavement. Edited by Stroebe MS, Stroebe W, Hansson R. Cambridge, United Kingdom, Cambridge University Press, 1993, pp 397–410

Viney L: The construing widow: dislocation and adaptation in bereavement. Psychotherapy Patient 6:207–222, 1990

Chapter 22

Sleep and Circadian Rhythm Disorders

Select the single best response for each question.

22.1 Extensive research has shown that marked changes in sleep and circadian rhythms accompany aging. Which of the following is an example of the changes that will occur with aging?

    A. Nocturnal sleep time increases.
    B. Time in stages 3 and 4 sleep increases.
    C. Nocturnal wake time increases.
    D. The amplitude of the sleep-wake cycle increases.
    E. Older adults tend to awaken at a later phase.

The correct response is option C.

Nocturnal sleep time steadily decreases across the life span, and nocturnal wake time increases, because of an increase in arousals. Accompanying these changes are marked reductions in stages 3 and 4 sleep (these stages are the deeper stages of non–rapid eye movement [NREM] sleep). Although the clinical significance of these changes is unknown, they may relate to the reported reduction in subjective sleep quality and lowering of the arousal threshold with age (Riedel and Lichstein 1998; Zepelin et al. 1984). The sleep-wake cycle appears to change significantly with age as well. The amplitudes of both the sleep-wake cycle and the 24-hour body temperature rhythm appear to decrease with aging (Bliwise 2000; Czeisler et al. 1999). Additionally, compared with younger age groups, older adults tend to awaken at an earlier phase (i.e., closer to the nadir of their 24-hour temperature rhythms), and they show a greater propensity to awaken during the later portions of their sleep episodes (Dijk et al. 1997; Duffy et al. 1998). **(p. 396)**

22.2 Which of the following primary sleep disorders is rare in adults age 60 years or older?

    A. Restless legs syndrome (RLS).
    B. Obstructive sleep apnea.
    C. Insomnia from depression.
    D. Periodic limb movement disorder (PLMD).
    E. Central sleep apnea.

The correct response is option E.

Central sleep apnea is relatively rare, constituting 4%–10% of patients with apnea (White 2000). The predominant type of sleep apnea seen in elderly individuals is obstructive sleep apnea (Ancoli-Israel et al. 1987). A number of studies suggest that the frequency of obstructive sleep apnea increases with age (Ancoli-Israel 1989; Ancoli-Israel et al. 1991; Dickel and Mosko 1990; Roehrs et al. 1983).

    RLS occurs in 6% of the adult population and is present in up to 28% of patients older than 65 years (Clark 2001).

Depression is frequently associated with sleep disruption in individuals older than age 60. Roughly 10%–15% of individuals older than 65 years experience clinically significant depressive symptoms (Hoch et al. 1989). The most frequent complaints in affected individuals are 1) a decrease in total sleep time and 2) waking earlier than desired. Daytime sleepiness may occur but is less common.

Several studies indicate that clinically significant PLMD is seen in 30%–45% of adults age 60 years or older, compared with 5%–6% of all adults (Ancoli-Israel et al. 1991). **(pp. 397, 398)**

22.3   Individuals with Alzheimer's disease experience a number of sleep changes. Which of the following is among the leading reasons that individuals with dementia become institutionalized?

    A. Increased arousals.
    B. Sundowning.
    C. More daytime naps.
    D. Decreased REM sleep.
    E. Decreased slow wave sleep.

The correct response is option B.

Individuals with dementia often experience evening or nocturnal agitation and confusion. This phenomenon, called *sundowning,* is among the leading reasons that individuals with dementia become institutionalized (Pollak and Perlick 1991; Pollak et al. 1990; Sanford 1975).

Individuals with Alzheimer's disease have been found to experience an increased number of arousals and awakenings, to take more daytime naps, and to have a diminished amount of REM sleep and slow-wave sleep (Prinz et al. 1982). **(p. 399)**

22.4   The most troublesome symptom of sleep disturbance for patients with Parkinson's disease is

    A. Difficulty initiating sleep.
    B. Restless legs syndrome.
    C. Daytime fatigue.
    D. Difficulty maintaining sleep.
    E. Inability to turn over in bed.

The correct response is option E.

Sleep complaints are noted in 60%–90% of individuals with Parkinson's disease (Trenkwalder 1998). The majority of Parkinson's disease patients with affected sleep experience difficulty in initiating and maintaining sleep, daytime fatigue, RLS, and an inability to turn over in bed. The last of these features was rated as the most troublesome symptom of sleep disturbance in a study by Lees et al. (1988). **(p. 399)**

22.5   Individuals with chronic obstructive pulmonary disease (COPD) have been found to have evidence of disturbed sleep. Which of the following statements concerning COPD and sleep is true?

    A. Daytime sleepiness does not routinely occur in COPD.
    B. Polysomnography is routinely indicated for COPD patients.
    C. The degree of sleep disturbance in COPD patients is related to the degree of hypoxemia.
    D. COPD patients who become hypoxemic at night are less likely to be hypoxemic during the day.
    E. Sleep apnea is more common in COPD patients than in the general population.

The correct response is option A.

Individuals with COPD have been found to have both subjective and objective evidence of disturbed sleep, but the degree of sleep disruption is unrelated to hypoxemia (Douglas 2000). Also, daytime sleepiness, which is seen in patients with sleep apnea, does not appear to occur. Polysomnography is not routinely indicated for individuals with COPD who have sleep difficulties (Connaughton et al. 1988), and the need for polysomnography in COPD patients should be determined in the same way that the need in other patients is determined. Sleep apnea appears to be no more common in persons with COPD than in the general population. Nocturnal oxygen may be needed in some patients; however, patients who tend to become most hypoxemic at night are patients who are most hypoxemic during the day (Connaughton et al. 1988). **(p. 400)**

22.6   The most common reason given by elderly persons for difficulty in maintaining sleep is

    A. Restless legs syndrome.
    B. Depression.
    C. Periodic limb movement.
    D. Nocturia.
    E. Daytime naps.

The correct response is option D.

The urge to urinate is an often overlooked cause of awakenings in the elderly population (Bliwise 2000). Surprisingly, it has been reported that nocturia (excessive urination at night) is the most common explanation given by elderly individuals for difficulty in maintaining sleep; 63%–72% of elderly persons cite nocturia as a reason for sleep maintenance problems (Middelkoop et al. 1996). Furthermore, several studies have documented the sleep disturbance caused by and daytime adverse effects of nocturia (Bliwise 2000). The most common causes of nocturia are conditions that increase in frequency with age: benign prostatic hypertrophy in men and decreased urethral resistance due to decreased estrogen levels in women (Bliwise 2000). **(p. 400)**

22.7   You evaluate an elderly patient for depression and decide to begin her on an antidepressant because a significant problem for her has been sleep difficulties. She reports that she is able to fall asleep quickly, but that she awakens throughout the night. Which of the following agents would improve her ability to stay asleep?

    A. Ramelteon.
    B. Zaleplon.
    C. Eszopiclone.
    D. Zolpidem.
    E. Amitriptyline.

The correct response is option C.

Of the agents available in the United States, eszopiclone is the only one demonstrated to improve the ability to stay asleep in older adults with insomnia (McCall et al. 2006). A number of the benzodiazepines have half-lives that are so long that they are unsuitable insomnia agents because of inevitable daytime impairment. Only triazolam and temazepam have half-lives in the range such that they are reasonable to use in the treatment of insomnia.

Of the medications most frequently used to treat insomnia, the nonbenzodiazepine hypnotic zaleplon and the melatonin-receptor agonist ramelteon have the shortest half-lives (approximately 1 hour), making them well suited for treating problems falling asleep. Because of its short half-life, zaleplon may also be useful in the middle of the night for individuals who sometimes wake up at that time (Stone et al. 2002).

Zolpidem, with a half-life of approximately 2.5 hours, is another agent approved for the treatment of difficulties in falling asleep. Although the agent with the shortest half-life that effectively treats the sleep difficulty should always be used in order to minimize risks, individuals with difficulty staying asleep generally will need longer-acting agents.

Although antidepressants are widely used to treat insomnia in the United States (most notably trazodone, mirtazapine, doxepin, and amitriptyline), there has yet to be a study of any of these agents in older adults with insomnia (Walsh 2004). **(p. 404)**

References

Ancoli-Israel S: Epidemiology of sleep disorders. Clin Geriatr Med 5:347–362, 1989

Ancoli-Israel S, Kripke DF, Mason W: Characteristics of obstructive and central sleep apnea in the elderly: an interim report. Biol Psychiatry 22:741–750, 1987

Ancoli-Israel S, Kripke DF, Klauber MR, et al: Periodic limb movements in sleep in community-dwelling elderly. Sleep 14:496–500, 1991

Bliwise DL: Normal aging, in Principles and Practice of Sleep Medicine, 3rd Edition. Edited by Kryger MH, Roth T, Dement WC. Philadelphia, PA, WB Saunders, 2000, pp 26–42

Clark MM: Restless legs syndrome. J Am Board Fam Pract 14:368–374, 2001

Connaughton JJ, Catterall JR, Elton RA, et al: Do sleep studies contribute to the management of patients with severe chronic obstructive pulmonary disease? Am Rev Respir Dis 138:341–344, 1988

Czeisler CA, Duffy JF, Shanahan TL, et al: Stability, precision, and near-24-hour period of the human circadian pacemaker. Science 284:2177–2181, 1999

Dickel MJ, Mosko SS: Morbidity cut-offs for sleep apnea and periodic leg movements in predicting subjective complaints in seniors. Sleep 13:155–166, 1990

Dijk DJ, Duffy JF, Riel E, et al: Altered interaction of circadian and homeostatic aspects of sleep propensity results in awakening at an earlier circadian phase in older people. Sleep Research 26:710, 1997

Douglas NJ: Chronic obstructive pulmonary disease, in Principles and Practice of Sleep Medicine, 3rd Edition. Edited by Kryger MH, Roth T, Dement WC. Philadelphia, PA, WB Saunders, 2000, pp 965–975

Duffy JF, Dijk DJ, Klerman EB, et al: Later endogenous circadian temperature nadir relative to an earlier wake time in older people. Am J Physiol 275:R1478–R1487, 1998

Hoch CC, Buysse DJ, Reynolds CF: Sleep and depression in late life. Clin Geriatr Med 5:259–272, 1989

Lees AJ, Blackburn NA, Campbell VL: The nighttime problems of Parkinson's disease. Clin Neuropharmacol 11:512–519, 1988

McCall WV, Erman M, Krystal AD, et al: A polysomnography study of eszopiclone in elderly patients with insomnia. Curr Med Res Opin 22:1633–1642, 2006

Middelkoop HA, Smilde-van den Doel DA, Neven AK, et al: Subjective sleep characteristics of 1,485 males and females aged 50–93: effects of sex and age and factors related to self-evaluated quality of sleep. J Gerontol A Biol Sci Med Sci 51:M108–M115, 1996

Pollak CP, Perlick D, Lisner JP, et al: Sleep problems in the community elderly as predictors of death and nursing home placement. J Community Health 15:123–135, 1990

Pollak CP, Perlick D: Sleep problems and institutionalization of the elderly. J Geriatr Psychiatry Neurol 4:204–210, 1991

Prinz PN, Peskind ER, Vitaliano PP, et al: Changes in the sleep and waking EEGs of nondemented and demented elderly subjects. J Am Geriatr Soc 30:86–93, 1982

Riedel BW, Lichstein KL: Objective sleep measures and subjective sleep satisfaction: how do older adults with insomnia define a good night's sleep? Psychol Aging 13:159–163, 1998

Roehrs T, Zorick F, Sicklesteel J, et al: Age-related sleep-wake disorders at a sleep disorder center. J Am Geriatr Soc 31:364–370, 1983

Sanford JR: Tolerance of debility in elderly dependants by supporters at home: its significance for hospital practice. Br Med J 3:471–473, 1975

Stone BM, Turner C, Mills SL, et al: Noise-induced sleep maintenance insomnia: hypnotic and residual effects of zaleplon. Br J Clin Pharmacol 53:196–202, 2002

Trenkwalder C: Sleep dysfunction in Parkinson's disease. Clin Neurosci 5:107–114, 1998

Walsh JK: Drugs used to treat insomnia in 2002: regulatory-based rather than evidence-based medicine. Sleep 27:14441–14442, 2004

White DP: Central sleep apnea, in Principles and Practice of Sleep Medicine, 3rd Edition. Edited by Kryger MH, Roth T, Dement WC. Philadelphia, WB Saunders, 2000, pp 827–839

Zepelin H, McDonald CS, Zammit GK: Effects of age on auditory awakening thresholds. J Gerontol 39:294–300, 1984

Chapter 23

Alcohol and Drug Problems

Select the single best response for each question.

23.1 When consumption of alcohol is at a level whereby adverse medical, psychological, or social consequences have occurred, older adults would be characterized as

A. Alcohol dependent.
B. Low-risk drinkers.
C. Problem users.
D. At-risk drinkers.
E. Abstainers.

The correct response is option C.

When consumption of alcohol or drugs is at a level whereby adverse medical, psychological, or social consequences have occurred or are significantly likely to occur, older adults are said to follow a pattern of *problem use or abuse.*

According to DSM-IV-TR criteria, *alcohol or drug dependence* is defined as a medical disorder marked by clinically significant distress or impairment coupled with preoccupation with alcohol or drugs, loss of control, continued substance use despite adverse consequences, and/or physiological symptoms such as tolerance and withdrawal (American Psychiatric Association 2000) (Table 23–1).

Low-risk, social, or moderate drinkers include individuals who drink within the recommended guidelines (i.e., drink no more than one drink per day) and do not exhibit any alcohol-related problems. Older adults in this group also observe caution and do not drink when driving a motor vehicle or boat, nor do they drink when using contraindicated medications.

Older adults who consume substances above recommended levels yet experience minimal or no substance-related health, social, or emotional problems represent *at-risk or excessive substance users.* At-risk substance use generally applies to the consumption of alcohol or prescription and over-the-counter medications rather than illicit drugs.

Individuals who report drinking less than 1–2 drinks in the previous year are described as *abstainers.* This is the most common drinking pattern in later life, with approximately 50%–70% of older adults reporting abstinence (Blow 1998; Kirchner et al. 2007). **(pp. 411–413)**

23.2 All of the following are beneficial effects of moderate alcohol consumption *except*

A. Reduced risk of cardiovascular disease.
B. Reduced risk of diabetes.
C. Improved self-esteem.
D. Lower odds of reporting physical limitations.
E. Lower high-density lipoprotein serum level.

The correct response is option E.

TABLE 23–1. DSM-IV-TR criteria for substance abuse and dependence

Criteria for Substance Abuse

A. A maladaptive pattern of substance use leading to clinically significant impairment or distress, as manifested by one (or more) of the following, occurring within a 12-month period:

    (1) recurrent substance use resulting in a failure to fulfill major role obligations at work, school, or home (e.g., repeated absences or poor work performance related to substance use; substance-related absences, suspensions, or expulsions from school; neglect of children or household)

    (2) recurrent substance use in situations in which it is physically hazardous (e.g., driving an automobile or operating a machine when impaired by substance use)

    (3) recurrent substance-related legal problems (e.g., arrests for substance-related disorderly conduct)

    (4) continued substance use despite having persistent or recurrent social or interpersonal problems caused or exacerbated by the effects of the substance (e.g., arguments with spouse about consequences of intoxication, physical fights)

B. The symptoms have never met the criteria for Substance Dependence for this class of substance.

Criteria for Substance Dependence

A maladaptive pattern of substance use, leading to clinically significant impairment or distress, as manifested by three (or more) of the following, occurring at any time in the same 12-month period:

    (1) tolerance, as defined by either of the following:

        (a) a need for markedly increased amounts of the substance to achieve intoxication or desired effect

        (b) markedly diminished effect with continued use of the same amount of the substance

    (2) withdrawal, as manifested by either of the following:

        (a) the characteristic withdrawal syndrome for the substance (refer to Criteria A and B of the criteria sets for withdrawal from the specific substances)

        (b) the same (or a closely related) substance is taken to relieve or avoid withdrawal symptoms

    (3) the substance is often taken in larger amounts or over a longer period than was intended

    (4) there is a persistent desire or unsuccessful efforts to cut down or control substance use

    (5) a great deal of time is spent in activities necessary to obtain the substance (e.g., visiting multiple doctors or driving long distances), use the substance (e.g., chain-smoking), or recover from its effects

    (6) important social, occupational, or recreational activities are given up or reduced because of substance use

    (7) the substance use is continued despite knowledge of having a persistent or recurrent physical or psychological problem that is likely to have been caused or exacerbated by the substance (e.g., current cocaine use despite recognition of cocaine-induced depression, or continued drinking despite recognition that an ulcer was made worse by alcohol consumption)

Specify if:

With Physiological Dependence: evidence of tolerance or withdrawal (i.e., either Item 1 or 2 is present)

Without Physiological Dependence: no evidence of tolerance or withdrawal (i.e., neither Item 1 nor 2 is present)

Course specifiers (see text for definitions):

Early Full Remission

Early Partial Remission

Sustained Full Remission

Sustained Partial Remission

On Agonist Therapy

In a Controlled Environment

Source. Reprinted from *Diagnostic and Statistical Manual of Mental Disorders*, 4th Edition, Text Revision. Washington, DC, American Psychiatric Association, 2000. Copyright 2000, American Psychiatric Association. Used with permission.

There is some evidence to suggest that low-risk or moderate alcohol consumption may have a positive impact on physical health and mental well-being. For example, low-risk or moderate alcohol consumption is associated with a reduced risk of cardiovascular disease in both men and women and a reduced risk of cardiovascular disease–related disability (Rimm et al. 1991; Stampfer et al. 1988). Furthermore, researchers in one study of older adults without cardiovascular disease found that moderate alcohol consumption was related to lipoprotein subclass distribution (Mukamal et al. 2007). Specifically, results indicated that moderate alcohol use was associated with fewer small low-density lipoprotein particles and a greater number of large- and medium-sized high-density lipoprotein (HDL) particles. In their prospective study of 4,655 older adults with no diabetes at baseline, Djousse et al. (2007) found that regardless of the type of beverage consumed, light to moderate alcohol consumption was associated with a lower incidence of diabetes approximately 6.3 years later. With respect to functional decline, findings from cross-sectional work suggest that among older men, low to moderate alcohol consumption is associated with lower odds of reporting physical limitations when compared with abstinence or heavy use (Cawthon et al. 2007). Finally, light to moderate alcohol use has beneficial effects on subjective well-being for both men and women (Lang et al. 2007) and improves self-esteem, reduces stress, and provides relaxation, particularly in social situations (Dufour et al. 1992). **(pp. 415–416)**

23.3 For a number of reasons, providers may fail to identify alcohol and substance use disorders in older patients. Which of the following is ***not*** one of the reasons for failure to identify these disorders?

    A. Mistaken belief that there are too many effective treatments.
    B. Misconception that older substance users must have a lifelong history of problem use.
    C. Difficulty in applying diagnostic criteria for substance use disorders to seniors.
    D. Lack of appreciation of the benefits of reduced substance use.
    E. Insufficient knowledge of the potential health impact of problem drinking.

The correct response is option A.

The belief that there are few accessible and effective treatments for substance use and a general lack of appreciation of the benefits of reduced substance use in the absence of abuse or dependence have the potential to significantly reduce a clinician's motivation to screen for or recognize at-risk or problem drinking.

At the provider level, the common misconception that older substance users have a lifelong history of problem use may make it difficult for clinicians to identify individuals who either have late-onset conditions or are at high risk for them. Furthermore, insufficient knowledge regarding symptoms or the potential health impact of at-risk or problematic drinking may inhibit screening efforts. Diagnostic criteria and symptoms for alcohol and prescription drug misuse are not easily applied to older adults and are often confounded with symptoms of comorbid medical illnesses, further complicating the screening and diagnostic process for providers. Additionally, the use of multiple diagnostic terms can lead to confusion as to who should be screened, how screening should proceed, and which problems or patterns of use should be treated. **(p. 417)**

23.4 The "gold standard" for assessing the quantity and frequency of alcohol and drug use is

    A. The timeline follow-back method (TLFB).
    B. Questions regarding average consumption practices.
    C. Prospective method.
    D. Retrospective diary method.
    E. Brown bag approach.

The correct response is option C.

Techniques used to assess the quantity and frequency of alcohol and drug use fall into one of three categories: questions regarding average consumption practices, retrospective accounts of daily use over some defined period of time (i.e., the TLFB), and prospective monitoring and recording of alcohol and drug use. The prospective diary method is considered to be the gold standard because it elicits the greatest amount of reports of consumption and is highly associated with sales data for alcoholic beverages among younger adults (Lemmens et al. 1992). Nevertheless, given the fact that proper completion of this type of measure is time consuming and requires multiple visits, this method is impractical for screening or brief assessments. The "brown bag approach," in which patients are asked to bring in all prescribed and over-the-counter medications they are currently taking, is a useful and convenient aid for determining medication use and misuse. **(p. 418)**

23.5 The timeline follow-back method is a commonly used technique for recording alcohol use in studies of addiction. A major limitation is

    A. It may overestimate use for less frequent users of alcohol.
    B. It is poorly correlated with reports from prospective diaries.
    C. It is less accurate when administered by an interviewer.
    D. The week being measured may not be representative of the person's usual drinking behavior.
    E. It may be administered more quickly than assessments of average alcohol frequency usage.

The correct response is option D.

The TLFB method represents the most commonly used technique in treatment studies for addiction and has become the standard method of choice for such studies. Among older adults, 7-day TLFB assessments are highly correlated with reports from prospective diaries. Nevertheless, certain difficulties arise when using this method. First, the specific week of measurement under assessment may not be representative of the individual's usual drinking behavior. Second, although the TLFB closely matches prospective diary reports for nondrinkers or daily drinkers, it underestimates use for less frequent users of alcohol (Lemmens et al. 1992). The TLFB also takes longer to administer than measures assessing average frequency, and because of variation in individuals' definitions of a "standard" drink, it is more effective and accurate when administered by an interviewer as opposed to self-administration. **(p. 418)**

23.6 Which of the following is a long-term marker of alcohol use?

    A. Gamma-glutamyl transferase (GGT).
    B. Hematocrit.
    C. Blood urea nitrogen.
    D. Low-density lipoprotein level.
    E. Serum bilirubin.

The correct response is option A.

Long-term markers of alcohol use include GGT, mean corpuscular volume, high-density lipoprotein level, and carbohydrate-deficient transferrin (Oslin et al. 1998). **(p. 420)**

23.7 In 1995 the U.S. Food and Drug Administration (FDA) approved the first medication in over 50 years for the treatment of alcohol dependence. Which of the following is the medication?

    A. Disulfiram.
    B. Naltrexone.
    C. Naloxone.
    D. Acamprosate.
    E. Bupropion.

The correct response is option B.

In 1995, the opioid antagonist naltrexone became the first pharmacological agent approved by the FDA in over 50 years for use in the treatment of alcohol dependence. Approval of the drug was based on findings from clinical trials that showed that naltrexone was safe and effective in preventing relapse and reducing alcohol cravings (O'Malley et al. 1992; Volpicelli et al. 1992).

Until recently, the long-term treatment of older alcohol-dependent adults did not involve the use of pharmacological agents. Although disulfiram was originally the only medication approved for the treatment of alcohol dependence, it was seldom used in older patients because of the potential for adverse effects.

Acamprosate has emerged as another promising agent in the treatment of alcohol dependence. Although the exact action of acamprosate is still unclear, it is believed to reduce glutamate response (Pelc et al. 1997). The clinical evidence favoring acamprosate is impressive. **(p. 422)**

References

American Psychiatric Association: Diagnostic and Statistical Manual of Mental Disorders, 4th Edition, Text Revision. Washington, DC, American Psychiatric Association, 2000

Blow FC (Consensus Panel Chair): Substance Abuse Among Older Adults. Treatment Improvement Series Protocol (TIP) Series No. 26. Center for Substance Abuse Treatment. Rockville, MD, U.S. Department of Health and Human Services, 1998

Cawthon PM, Fink HA, Barrett-Connor E, et al: Alcohol use, physical performance, and functional limitations in older men. J Am Geriatr Soc 55:212–220, 2007

Djousse L, Biggs ML, Mukamal KJ, et al: Alcohol consumption and type 2 diabetes among older adults: the cardiovascular health study. Obesity 15:1758–1765, 2007

Dufour MC, Archer L, Gordis E: Alcohol and the elderly. Clin Geriatr Med 8:127–141, 1992

Kirchner JE, Zubritsky C, Cody M, et al: Alcohol consumption among older adults in primary care. J Gen Intern Med 22:92–97, 2007

Lang I, Wallace RB, Huppert FA, et al: Moderate alcohol consumption in older adults is associated with better cognition and well-being than abstinence. Age and Ageing 36:256–261, 2007

Lemmens P, Tan ES, Knibbe RA: Measuring quantity and frequency of drinking in a general population survey: a comparison of five indices. J Stud Alcohol 53:476–486, 1992

Mukamal KJ, Mackey RH, Kuller LH, et al: Alcohol consumption and lipoprotein subclasses in older adults. J Clin Endocrinol Metab 92:2559–2566, 2007

O'Malley SS, Jaffe AJ, Chang G, et al: Naltrexone and coping skills therapy for alcohol dependence: a controlled study. Arch Gen Psychiatry 49:881–887, 1992

Oslin DW, Pettinati HM, Luck G, et al: Clinical correlations with carbohydrate-deficient transferrin levels in women with alcoholism. Alcohol Clin Exp Res 22:1981–1985, 1998

Pelc I, Verbanck P, Le Bon O, et al: Efficacy and safety of acamprosate in the treatment of detoxified alcohol-dependent patients: a 90-day placebo-controlled dose-finding study. Br J Psychiatry 171:73–77, 1997

Rimm EB, Giovannucci EL, Willett WC, et al: Prospective study of alcohol consumption and risk of coronary disease in men. Lancet 338:464–468, 1991

Stampfer MJ, Colditz GA, Willett WC, et al: A prospective study of moderate alcohol consumption and the risk of coronary disease and stroke in women. N Engl J Med 319:267–273, 1988

Volpicelli JR, Alterman AI, Hayashida M, et al: Naltrexone in the treatment of alcohol dependence. Arch Gen Psychiatry 49:876–880, 1992

Personality Disorders

Select the single best response for each question.

24.1 You are asked to evaluate a 75-year-old woman who was referred by her internist. She exhibits the following long-standing characteristics: sensitivity to rejection and chronic feelings of abandonment. You suspect that she has a personality disorder. Which of the following personality disorders is most likely?

    A. Avoidant.
    B. Borderline.
    C. Dependent.
    D. Paranoid.
    E. Schizoid.

The correct response is option B.

Since 1980, DSM has categorized three different personality disorder clusters: A—odd, eccentric (including paranoid, schizoid, and schizotypal personality disorders); B—dramatic, erratic (including borderline, histrionic, narcissistic, and antisocial personality disorders); and C—anxious, fearful (including obsessive-compulsive, avoidant, and dependent personality disorders). Borderline patients are quite sensitive to rejection and have long-standing feelings of abandonment. Patients with avoidant personality exhibit the key characteristics of vulnerability and inhibition. Dependent personality disorder is characterized by helplessness and overattachment. Seniors with paranoid personality disorder view people as dangerous; consequently, they are vigilant and suspicious. Finally, patients with schizoid personality disorder exhibit isolation and autonomy. **(pp. 430–431)**

24.2 Which of the following statements concerning personality disorders in seniors is *false*?

    A. The prevalence of personality disorders in older persons is generally twice the rate of personality disorders in younger persons in the general population.
    B. The single most common comorbid Axis I condition in seniors with personality disorders is depression.
    C. The prevalence of personality disorders in selected outpatient or inpatient samples of older persons can be as high as 25%–65%.
    D. The prevalence of personality disorders in the general population is estimated at 10%–15% of all ages.
    E. The prevalence of personality disorders in psychiatric settings is usually three to four times higher than in the community.

The correct response is option A.

The prevalence of personality disorders in older persons generally is lower by about half than that in younger persons in the general population (i.e., 5%–10%). The prevalence in selected outpatient or inpatient samples of older persons can be as high as 25%–65% (Agbayewa 1996; Agronin and Maletta 2000; Ames and Molinari 1994; Camus et al. 1997; Cohen et al. 1994; Fogel and Westlake 1990; Kenan et al. 2000).

    The association of personality disorders with depressive disorders in the elderly population is probably the single most reported comorbidity—especially Cluster C avoidant and dependent personality disorders (Abrams et al. 1994; Agbayewa 1996; Camus et al. 1997; Devanand et al. 2000; Fogel and Westlake 1990; Kunik et al. 1993; Morse and Lynch 2004; Nubukpo et al. 2005), Cluster B personality disorders (Abrams et al. 2001; Sato et al. 1999; Vine and Steingart 1994), and personality disorder not otherwise specified (Kunik et al. 1993).

The prevalence of personality disorders in the general population is less accurately known than that of Axis I disorders but is estimated at 10%–15% for all ages (Agronin and Maletta 2000; Grant et al. 2004; Lenzenweger et al. 1997; Weissman 1990), a relatively high rate compared with many Axis I disorders. The prevalence of personality disorders in psychiatric settings is usually three to four times higher than that in the community, with frequent comorbidity of Axis I and Axis II disorders (Kunik et al. 1994; Zweig and Hillman 1999). **(pp. 430–431)**

24.3 Both Erikson and Vaillant studied late-life development. All of the following statements concerning their work are true *except*

A. Mature defenses were more consistently identified in Erickson's later developmental stages.
B. Erikson proposed that the major developmental task of older age is to look back and seek meaning across the life span.
C. An example of a mature and adaptive defense mechanism is suppression.
D. Mature defenses are dependent upon education and social privilege.
E. Mature defenses synthesize and attenuate conflicts.

The correct response is option D.

Across several longitudinal studies that included privileged persons (Heath 1945), gifted persons (Terman 1925), and persons from the core inner cities (Glueck and Glueck 1968), Vaillant established that mature defenses were more consistently identified primarily in Erikson's later developmental stages (Vaillant 1993; Vaillant and Drake 1985) and that the development of these defenses was independent of education and social privilege (Vaillant 1993).

Erikson's stage theory of late-life development (Erikson et al. 1986) proposed that the major developmental task of older age is to look back and seek meaning across the life span, rather than looking forward, as in previous developmental modes that are now in decline. The goal of this task as discussed by Erikson is to maintain more integrity than despair about one's life.

Vaillant and others (e.g., Diehl et al. 1996) have provided empirical verification for Erikson's life-stage concepts through longitudinal study of the maturation of defenses across the life span (Vaillant 2000, 2002; Vaillant and Milofsky 1980). Defenses are involuntary mental mechanisms for regulating the realities that persons are powerless to change. Vaillant and others (Haan 1977) have described a hierarchy of defenses from immature and maladaptive to mature and adaptive. Mature defenses include humor, altruism, sublimation, anticipation, and suppression. Mature and adaptive defenses synthesize and attenuate conflicts rather than distorting or denying them. **(pp. 432–433)**

24.4 You are asked by a colleague to evaluate an 80-year-old man for a possible personality disorder. You want to use a reliable and valid dimensional assessment tool that has proved useful as a screening tool in the elderly. Which of the following instruments would you select?

A. Millon Clinical Multiaxial Inventory—III (MCMI-III).
B. Personality Diagnostic Questionnaire (PDQ-IV).
C. Schedule for Nonadaptive and Adaptive Personality.
D. Wisconsin Personality Disorders Inventory.
E. The Neuroticism, Extraversion, Openness Five Factor Model (NEO-FFM).

The correct response is option E.

Several ancillary self-report instruments are available for initial screening purposes—e.g., the MCMI-III (Millon 1994), PDQ-IV (Hyler et al. 1988), Schedule for Nonadaptive and Adaptive Personality (Clark 1993), and Wisconsin Personality Disorders Inventory (Klein et al. 1993). However, the results of these self-reports have a low concordance with the results of interview methods (Perry 1992), and their use is best established and tolerated in younger populations, not among elders, in whom acquired brain disease is an increasing issue. The NEO-FFM (Costa and McCrae 1985, 1997) is a reliable and valid dimensional assessment tool for personality traits that has been used with the elderly. It has also proved useful as a screening tool for personality disorders (Miller et al. 2005). **(pp. 433–434)**

24.5 A 75-year-old woman whom you are called by a neurologist to evaluate was noted to have frontal lobe damage due to a motor vehicle accident. In evaluating her, you note many difficulties similar to which of the following personality disorders?

  A. Avoidant.
  B. Borderline.
  C. Dependent.
  D. Obsessive-compulsive.
  E. Schizotypal.

The correct response is option B.

Syndromes based on frontal lobe pathology that result in loss of normal executive function present some of the most difficult diagnostic challenges—especially if the onset of symptoms is subtle, the rate of progression is slow, and the main attributes of the premorbid personality are obscure. Patients with frontal or frontotemporal lobe disease may show good preservation of memory function. They are, however, prone to trouble with "mechanistic planning, verbal reasoning, or problem solving" and "obeying the rules of interpersonal social behavior, the experience of reward and punishment, and the interpretation of complex emotions" (Grafman and Litvan 1999, p. 1921; Passant et al. 2005). These difficulties are similar to some of the problems experienced by many people with borderline, narcissistic, histrionic, paranoid, and antisocial personality disorders. **(p. 434)**

References

Abrams RC, Rosendahl E, Card C, et al: Personality disorder correlates of late and early onset depression. J Am Geriatr Soc 42:727–731, 1994

Abrams RC, Alexopoulos GS, Spielman LA, et al: Personality disorder symptoms predict declines in global functioning and quality of life in elderly depressed patients. Am J Geriatr Psychiatry 9:67–71, 2001

Agbayewa MO: Occurrence and effects of personality disorders in depression: are they the same in the old and young? Can J Psychiatry 41:223–226, 1996

Agronin ME, Maletta G: Personality disorders in late life: understanding and overcoming the gap in research. Am J Geriatr Psychiatry 8:4–18, 2000

Ames A, Molinari V: Prevalence of personality disorders in community-living elderly. J Geriatr Psychiatry Neurol 7:189–194, 1994

Camus V, De Mendonca Lima CA, Gaillard M, et al: Are personality disorders more frequent in early onset geriatric depression? J Affect Disord 46:297–302, 1997

Clark LA: Manual for the Schedule for Nonadaptive and Adaptive Personality (SNAP). Minneapolis, MN, University of Minnesota Press, 1993

Cohen BJ, Nestadt G, Samuels JF, et al: Personality disorder in later life: a community study. Br J Psychiatry 165:493–499, 1994

Costa PT, McCrae RR: The NEO Personality Inventory Manual. Odessa, FL, Psychological Assessment Resources, 1985

Costa PT Jr, McCrae RR: Stability and change in personality assessment: the revised NEO Personality Inventory in the year 2000. J Pers Assess 68:86–94, 1997

Devanand DP, Turret N, Moody BJ, et al: Personality disorders in elderly patients with dysthymic disorder. Am J Geriatr Psychiatry 8:188–195, 2000

Diehl M, Coyle N, Labouvie-Vief G: Age and sex differences in strategies of coping and defense across the life span. Psychol Aging 11:127–136, 1996

Erikson EH, Erikson JM, Kivnick HQ: Vital Involvement in Old Age. New York, WW Norton, 1986

Fogel BS, Westlake R: Personality disorder diagnoses and age in inpatients with major depression. J Clin Psychiatry 51:232–235, 1990

Glueck S, Glueck E: Delinquents and Non-Delinquents in Perspective. Cambridge, MA, Harvard University Press, 1968

Grafman J, Litvan I: Importance of deficits in executive function. Lancet 354:1921–1922, 1999

Grant BF, Hasin DS, Stinson FS, et al: Prevalence, correlates, and disability of personality disorders in the United States: results from the national epidemiologic survey on alcohol and related conditions. J Clin Psychiatry 65:948–958, 2004

Haan NA: Coping and Defending. San Francisco, CA, Jossey-Bass, 1977

Heath C: What People Are. Cambridge, MA, Harvard University Press, 1945

Hyler SE, Rieder RO, Williams JBW, et al: The Personality Diagnostic Questionnaire: development and preliminary results. J Personal Disord 2:229–237, 1988

Kenan MM, Kendjelic EM, Molinari VA, et al: Age-related differences in the frequency of personality disorders among inpatient veterans. Int J Geriatr Psychiatry 15:831–837, 2000

Klein MH, Benjamin L, Rosenfelt R: The Wisconsin Personality Disorders Inventory. J Personal Disord 7:285–303, 1993

Kunik ME, Mulsant B, Rifai AH, et al: Personality disorders in elderly inpatients with major depression. Am J Geriatr Psychiatry 1:38–45, 1993

Kunik ME, Mulsant B, Rifai AH, et al: Diagnostic rate of comorbid personality disorder in elderly psychiatric inpatients. Am J Psychiatry 151:603–605, 1994

Lenzenweger MF, Loranger AW, Korfine L, et al: Detecting personality disorders in a nonclinical population: application for a two-stage procedure for case identification. Arch Gen Psychiatry 54:345–351, 1997

Miller JD, Bagby RM, Pilkonis PA, et al: A simplified technique for scoring DSM-IV personality disorders with the Five-Factor Model. Assessment 12:404–415, 2005

Millon T: Clinical Multiaxial Inventory—III (MCMI-III). Minneapolis, MN, National Computer Systems, 1994

Morse JQ, Lynch TR: A preliminary investigation of self-reported personality disorders in late life: prevalence, predictors of depressive severity, and clinical correlates. Aging Ment Health 8:307–315, 2004

Nubukpo P, Hartmann J, Clement JP: Role of personality in depression of the elderly: difference between early and late life depression. Psychol Neuropsychiatr Vieil 3:63–69, 2005

Passant U, Elfgren C, Englund E, et al: Psychiatric symptoms and their psychosocial consequences in frontotemporal dementia. Alzheimer Dis Assoc Disord 19 (suppl 1):S15–S18, 2005

Perry JC: Problems and considerations in the valid assessment of personality disorders. Am J Psychiatry 149:1645–1653, 1992

Sato T, Sakado K, Uehara T, et al: Personality disorder comorbidity in early-onset versus late-onset major depression in Japan. J Nerv Ment Dis 187:237–242, 1999

Terman LM: Genetic Studies of Genius, Vol 1: Mental and Physical Traits of a Thousand Gifted Children. Palo Alto, CA, Stanford University Press, 1925

Vaillant GE: The Wisdom of the Ego. Cambridge, MA, Harvard University Press, 1993

Vaillant GE: Adaptive mental mechanisms: their role in a positive psychology. Am Psychol 55:89–98, 2000

Vaillant GE: Aging Well. Boston, MA, Little, Brown, 2002

Vaillant GE, Drake RE: Maturity of ego defenses in relation to DSM-III axis II personality disorder. Arch Gen Psychiatry 42:597–601, 1985

Vaillant GE, Milofsky E: Natural history of male psychological health, IX: empirical evidence for Erikson's model of the life cycle. Am J Psychiatry 137:1348–1359, 1980

Vine RG, Steingart AB: Personality disorder in the elderly depressed. Can J Psychiatry 39:392–398, 1994

Weissman M: The epidemiology of personality disorders: a 1990 update. J Personal Disord 7 (suppl):44–62, 1990

Zweig R, Hillman J: Personality disorders in adults: a review, in Emerging Issues in Diagnosis and Treatment: LEA Series in Personality and Clinical Psychology. Edited by Rosowsky E, Abrams RC. Mahwah, NJ, Erlbaum, 1999, pp 31–53

Chapter 25

Agitation and Suspiciousness

Select the single best response for each question.

25.1 Kraepelin used the term *paraphrenia* to describe older patients who today would be most likely diagnosed according to DSM-IV-TR as having

A. Dementia.
B. Delirium.
C. Delusional disorder.
D. Schizoaffective disorder.
E. Bipolar I disorder.

The correct response is option C.

Among suspicious or paranoid elderly persons, one group has long been recognized, particularly in Europe. The term *late-life paraphrenia* has been used to identify psychosis that has a late age at onset and to distinguish the condition from both chronic schizophrenia and dementia. Kraepelin used *paraphrenia* to classify a small group of patients who exhibited paranoid delusions and yet were able to maintain functioning in their social milieu for months or years. He observed that persons with paraphrenia were typically women, usually living alone. Although current DSM diagnostic nomenclature would classify many of those individuals as having delusional disorder, this late-life syndrome may be more complex. **(p. 441)**

25.2 You ask the resident with whom you are working to outline some common nonpharmacological strategies for reducing agitation in an elderly patient whom you are treating. She comes up with the list below. You feel that all are good strategies *except*

A. Focusing the person's attention on the triggering event so they will gain more understanding.
B. Breaking down complex tasks into one-step guided directions.
C. Simplifying instructions.
D. Allowing adequate rest.
E. Providing pleasant distractions specific to the person.

The correct response is option A.

Nonpharmacological strategies for reducing agitation usually involve redirection of the person's attention away from triggering events or contexts or distraction with offers of pleasant events specific to the person (going out for ice cream or a ride, listening to favorite music, or watching old videotapes). Other strategies include breaking down complex tasks into one-step guided directions, simplifying instructions, and allowing adequate rest or passive observation between stimulating activities. **(p. 444)**

25.3 There are a number of communication strategies that may reduce a person's agitation. Which of the following is an example of one of these strategies?

    A. Avoid eye contact.
    B. Use popular expressions such as "don't go there."
    C. Ask the patient if he or she remembers you.
    D. Listen and don't feel compelled to talk constantly.
    E. Inquire as to what the patient wants to do, such as "Do you want to go now?"

The correct response is option D.

First it is necessary to get the person's attention. Make sure vision and hearing are adequate or "tuned up." Use eye contact, call the person by name in a clear, adult tone, approach slowly from the side or front or crouch down at his or her level, and offer your hand, palm up. Listen, but do not feel compelled to talk constantly. Words are not as important as a calm tone, a pleasant expression, and a nondistracting environment (turn off the TV or turn down the radio). Use familiar words, speak in a normal tone and tempo, but give the person time to process and respond. Repeat your words exactly, if necessary. Ask questions if you are unsure of his or her meaning ("Am I getting closer to what you want?"). Be patient—you may need to repeat to reassure him or her.

If frustration mounts, take a deep breath and suggest a better time to talk or another topic. Avoid popular expressions that may be ambiguous or vague, such as "Don't go there," "NOT," or "bottom line." Use concrete subjects, names, and references. Avoid pronouns. Do not test or ask the person if he or she remembers you. Use positive statements such as "Let's go," rather than "Do you want to go now?" Explain what happens next, but wait until just before it will happen. Demonstrate or model so that he or she can follow your lead. Use appropriate, respectful humor or his or her favorite phrases ("See ya later, alligator"). It is always appropriate to make fun of yourself, especially if you forget. Smile, nod, gesture, or use photos when words fail. **(p. 444)**

25.4 You are called to evaluate a patient with Parkinson's disease who has become psychotic and agitated. An especially effective agent is

    A. Haloperidol.
    B. Quetiapine.
    C. Lorazepam.
    D. Aripiprazole.
    E. Pimozide.

The correct response is option B.

If environmental measures are insufficient to control agitated or aggressive behavior, medication is usually needed. Guidelines for pharmacological treatment of agitation in elderly patients with dementia have been developed (Alexopoulos et al. 1998). High-potency neuroleptics (e.g., haloperidol) are effective for controlling acute agitation, especially when psychotic features are present (Small et al. 1997), but care needs to be taken with these agents given the increased risk of extrapyramidal symptoms (EPS) in elderly patients. Although there is no evidence to suggest that one neuroleptic agent is more effective than another, the atypical antipsychotics— clozapine (Clozaril), risperidone (Risperdal), olanzapine (Zyprexa), quetiapine (Seroquel), and ziprasidone (Geodon)—have a lesser frequency of EPS (e.g., parkinsonism, tardive dyskinesia) than high-potency typical neuroleptic agents. These medications (especially quetiapine) are particularly useful in patients with Parkinson's disease who become agitated or psychotic, because the selective dopaminergic blockade is less likely to interfere with dopamine's therapeutic effect on the basal ganglia. **(p. 447)**

25.5 When a patient is exhibiting agitation on a regular basis and neuroleptics are required, what is a good medication strategy to follow?

   A. Administer high doses of medication to treat specific episodes.
   B. Avoid high-potency agents such as haloperidol.
   C. Sedate the patient as much as possible.
   D. Use benzodiazepines in combination with neuroleptics.
   E. Administer low doses on a regular basis.

The correct response is option E.

In general, when agitation is a consistent problem and neuroleptic treatment is required, we recommend starting with a low-dose agent (e.g., 0.5 mg of haloperidol or 0.25–0.5 mg of risperidone) and administering it on a regular basis rather than attempting to treat specific episodes of agitation. Treating frequently-occurring agitation on an as-needed basis makes administering medication difficult, requires larger doses of medication for adequate control, and is likely to cause sedation and further clouding of thought. Benzodiazepines can also be used to treat anxiety or infrequent agitation, but they are less effective than other agents for long-term treatment because of already noted limitations. **(p. 447)**

References

Alexopoulos GS, Silver JM, Kahn DA, et al (eds): Agitation in Older Persons With Dementia: A Postgraduate Medicine Special Report (The Expert Consensus Guideline Series). New York, McGraw-Hill, 1998

Small GW, Rabins PV, Barry PP, et al: Diagnosis and treatment of Alzheimer disease and related disorders: consensus statement of the American Association for Geriatric Psychiatry, the Alzheimer's Association, and the American Geriatrics Society. JAMA 278:1363–1371, 1997

Chapter 26

Psychopharmacology

Select the single best response for each question.

26.1 Data show that all available selective serotonin reuptake inhibitors (SSRIs) have similar efficacy and tolerability in the treatment of depression in older adults; however, experts favor which of the following agents?

   A. Fluvoxamine.
   B. Paroxetine.
   C. Escitalopram.
   D. Fluoxetine.
   E. Duloxetine.

The correct response is option C.

Data show that all available SSRIs have similar efficacy and tolerability in the treatment of depression in younger (Kroenke et al. 2001) and in older adults (Schneider and Olin 1995; Solai et al. 2001). However, experts favor the use of citalopram, escitalopram, or sertraline over fluvoxamine, fluoxetine, or paroxetine (Alexopoulos et al. 2001; Mulsant et al. 2001). This preference is in large part because of the preferred drugs' favorable pharmacokinetic profiles (Table 26–1), their lower potential for clinically significant drug interactions (Table 26–2), and data suggesting their superiority in terms of cognitive improvement (Burrows et al. 2002; Doraiswamy et al. 2003; Furlan et al. 2001; Newhouse et al. 2000; Nyth and Gottfries 1990; Nyth et al. 1992). **(pp. 454, 456, 457)**

26.2 Which of the SSRIs needs to be administered twice a day in the elderly?

   A. Fluvoxamine.
   B. Paroxetine.
   C. Sertraline.
   D. Citalopram.
   E. Fluoxetine.

The correct response is option A.

All the SSRIs can be administered in a single daily dose except for fluvoxamine, which should be given in two divided doses (see Table 26–1). **(pp. 454, 456)**

26.3 SSRIs may produce all of the following adverse side effects *except*

   A. Increased risk of post-surgical bleeding.
   B. Extrapyramidal symptoms.
   C. Fragility fractures.
   D. Tachycardia.
   E. Gastrointestinal bleeding.

The correct response is option D.

In contrast to tricyclic antidepressants, SSRIs may directly affect platelet activation (Pollock et al. 2000), and data have demonstrated that use of SSRIs is associated with a small but significant increase in the risk of gastrointestinal or postsurgical bleeding (Dalton et al. 2006; Looper 2007). Because SSRIs may act synergistically with other medications that increase the risk of gastrointestinal bleeding, such as nonsteroidal anti-inflammatory drugs or low-dose aspirin, SSRIs should be used cautiously in older patients treated with these medications.

SSRIs can also be associated with bradycardia and should be started with caution in patients with low heart rates (e.g., patients taking β-blockers). They may also cause extrapyramidal symptoms in older patients, although this is not common (Mamo et al. 2000), and they are well tolerated by most patients with Parkinson's disease (Chen et al. 2007). The risk of falls and hip fracture unfortunately has not been shown to differ among different classes of antidepressants (Liu et al. 1998). There is also concern that chronic use of SSRIs may contribute to the risk of fragility-related fractures through direct effects on bone metabolism (Richards et al. 2007). **(pp. 455–456)**

TABLE 26–1.   Pharmacokinetic properties of selective serotonin reuptake inhibitors

	Half-life (days), including active metabolite(s)	Proportionality of dosage to plasma concentration	Risk of uncomfortable withdrawal symptoms	Age-related pharmacokinetic changes?	Efficacious dosage range in elderly (mg/day)[a]
Citalopram	1–3	Linear across therapeutic range	Low	Yes	20–40
Escitalopram	1–3	Linear across therapeutic range	Low	Yes	10–20
Fluoxetine	7–10	Nonlinear at higher dosages	Very low	Yes	20–40
Fluvoxamine	0.5–1	Nonlinear at higher dosages	Moderate	Yes	50–300
Paroxetine	1	Nonlinear at higher dosages	Moderate	Yes	20–40
Sertraline	1–3	Linear across therapeutic range	Low	No	50–200

[a]Starting dosage is typically half of the lower efficacious dosage; all the selective serotonin reuptake inhibitors can be administered in single daily doses except for fluvoxamine, which should be given in two divided doses.

TABLE 26–2.   Newer antidepressants' inhibition of cytochrome P450 (CYP) and potential for clinically significant drug-drug interactions

	CYP1A2	CYP2C9/2C19	CYP2D6	CYP3A4	Potential for clinically significant drug-drug interaction
Bupropion	0	0	++	0	Moderate
Citalopram	+	0	+	0	Low
Duloxetine	0	0	+	+	Low
Escitalopram	+	0	+	0	Low
Fluoxetine	+	++	+++	++	High
Fluvoxamine	+++	+++	+	++	High
Mirtazapine	0	0	0	+	Low
Nefazodone	0	+	0	+++	High
Paroxetine	+	+	+++	+	Moderate
Sertraline	+	+	+	+	Low
Venlafaxine	0	0	0	0	Low

Note.   0=minimal or no inhibition; +=mild inhibition; ++=moderate inhibition; +++=strong inhibition.

Source [see textbook reference section].   Belpaire et al. 1998; Brosen et al. 1993; Crewe et al. 1992; Ereshefsky and Dugan 2000; Gram et al. 1993; Greenblatt et al. 1998, 1999; Greene and Barbhaiya 1997; Hua et al. 2004; Iribarne et al. 1998; Jeppesen et al. 1996; Kashuba et al. 1998; Kobayashi et al. 1995; Kotlyar et al. 2005; Pollock 1999; Preskorn and Magnus 1994, 1997; Rasmussen et al. 1998; Rickels et al. 1998; Solai et al. 1997, 2002; Spina and Scordo 2002; von Moltke et al. 1995, 2001; Weigmann et al. 2001.

26.4 With regard to the newer, non-SSRI antidepressants, which of the following may be less safe than sertraline in a frail, elderly population?

    A. Bupropion.
    B. Duloxetine.
    C. Mirtazapine.
    D. Nefazodone.
    E. Venlafaxine.

The correct response is option E.

Only limited controlled data support the efficacy and safety of bupropion, duloxetine, mirtazapine, nefazodone, or venlafaxine in older patients. Nevertheless, because of their usually favorable side-effect profiles in younger patients and their various mechanisms of action, these drugs are the preferred alternatives in older patients who do not respond to or who cannot tolerate SSRIs (Alexopoulos et al. 2001). Still, controlled data suggest that venlafaxine may be less safe than sertraline in a frail elderly population, with no evidence of greater efficacy (Oslin et al. 2003). Thus, in the absence of systematic research in older patients, newer agents should be used cautiously (Oslin et al. 2003; Rabins and Lyketsos 2005). **(p. 456)**

26.5 Which of the following newer antidepressants should be avoided in psychotic patients or in agitated patients at risk for the development of psychiatric symptoms?

    A. Bupropion.
    B. Duloxetine.
    C. Mirtazapine.
    D. Nefazodone.
    E. Venlafaxine.

The correct response is option A.

In addition to the three small geriatric trials supporting its safety, controlled data on the use of bupropion in patients with heart disease (Kiev et al. 1994; Roose et al. 1991), in smokers (Tashkin et al. 2001), and in patients with neuropathic pain (Semenchuk et al. 2001) confirm clinical experience that bupropion is relatively well tolerated by medically ill patients. Bupropion is contraindicated in patients with seizure disorders or who are at risk for seizure disorders (e.g., poststroke patients); however, the sustained-release preparation of bupropion appears to be associated with a very low incidence of seizure, comparable with other antidepressants (Dunner et al. 1998). Bupropion has also been associated with the onset of psychosis in case reports (Howard and Warnock 1999), and it is prudent to avoid this medication in psychotic patients and in agitated patients at risk for the development of psychotic symptoms. The propensity of bupropion to induce psychosis in patients at risk has been attributed to its action on dopaminergic neurotransmission (Howard and Warnock 1999). **(p. 457)**

26.6 Which of the following antidepressants has been approved by the U.S. Food and Drug Administration (FDA) for the treatment of pain associated with diabetic neuropathy?

    A. Bupropion.
    B. Duloxetine.
    C. Mirtazapine.
    D. Nefazodone.
    E. Venlafaxine.

The correct response is option B.

Duloxetine is the newest antidepressant approved in the United States. Like venlafaxine, duloxetine is a dual serotonin-norepinephrine reuptake inhibitor (SNRI) (Chalon et al. 2003). Randomized, controlled trials in younger patients support its efficacy and tolerability in the treatment of major depression (Hudson et al. 2005; Kirwin and Goren 2005). It is also approved for the treatment of pain associated with diabetic neuropathy (Goldstein et al. 2005), and some data support its efficacy in the treatment of stress urinary incontinence (Mariappan et al. 2005). Published placebo-controlled data on duloxetine in the elderly have also found it to be efficacious in the treatment of depression and to alleviate associated pain symptoms (Nelson et al. 2005; Raskin et al. 2007). **(pp. 457–458)**

26.7   Concerns have been expressed about which of the following newer antidepressants' adverse effects on cognition and driving performance?

    A. Bupropion.
    B. Duloxetine.
    C. Mirtazapine.
    D. Nefazodone.
    E. Venlafaxine.

The correct response is option C.

Although mirtazapine has been used to treat depression in frail nursing home patients (Roose et al. 2003) and in older patients with dementia (Raji and Brady 2001), there are concerns about its impact on cognition. It has been shown to impair driving performance in two placebo- and active comparator–controlled trials in healthy volunteers (Ridout et al. 2003; Wingen et al. 2005) and to cause delirium in older patients with organic brain syndromes (Bailer et al. 2000). This deleterious impact on cognition is possibly because of mirtazapine's antihistaminergic and sedative effect. Other adverse effects of mirtazapine include weight gain with lipid increase (Nicholas et al. 2003), and neutropenia or even agranulocytosis (Hutchison 2001; Stimmel et al. 1997). Although these hematological adverse effects are very rare, they may occur more frequently in patients with compromised immune function (Stimmel et al. 1997). **(p. 459)**

26.8   Which of the following agents has been reported to increase the incidence of hepatic toxicity?

    A. Bupropion.
    B. Duloxetine.
    C. Mirtazapine.
    D. Nefazodone.
    E. Venlafaxine.

The correct response is option D.

Given the absence of any controlled trial in geriatric depression, mediocre outcomes in an open study (Saiz-Ruiz et al. 2002), and reports that the incidence of hepatic toxicity or even liver failure is 10- to 30-fold higher with nefazodone than with other antidepressants (Carvajal García-Pando et al. 2002; Lucena et al. 1999), nefazodone is very rarely used in older patients. **(p. 459)**

26.9 In Great Britain, the National Institute of Clinical Excellence has recommended that which of the following agents should not be prescribed to patients with preexisting heart disease?

    A. Bupropion.
    B. Duloxetine.
    C. Mirtazapine.
    D. Nefazodone.
    E. Venlafaxine.

The correct response is option E.

Venlafaxine is associated with adverse effects that can be linked to its action on the adrenergic system. Adverse effects usually seen with tricyclic antidepressants (TCAs) have been described, including dry mouth, constipation, urinary retention, increased ocular pressure, cardiovascular problems, and transient agitation (Aragona et al. 1998; Benazzi 1997). Most of these are usually benign, but cardiovascular adverse effects are of concern in the elderly. Most clinicians are aware that venlafaxine can cause hypertension, generally in a dose-dependent fashion (Thase 1998; Zimmer et al. 1997). It has also been associated with clinically significant hypotension, electrocardiographic changes, arrhythmia, and acute ischemia (Davidson et al. 2005; Johnson et al. 2006; Lessard et al. 1999; Reznik et al. 1999). In Great Britain, the recommendations of the National Institute for Clinical Excellence are that venlafaxine should not be prescribed to patients with preexisting heart disease, that an electrocardiogram should be obtained at baseline, and that blood pressure and cardiac functions should be monitored in those patients taking higher doses (National Collaborating Centre for Mental Health 2004). **(p. 460)**

26.10 If a TCA is to be prescribed to an older patient, which of the following agents is preferred?

    A. Amitriptyline.
    B. Clomipramine.
    C. Desipramine.
    D. Doxepin.
    E. Imipramine.

The correct response is option C.

When one needs to use a TCA in an older patient, the secondary amines desipramine and nortriptyline are preferred because of their lower propensity to cause orthostasis and falls, their linear pharmacokinetics, and their more modest anticholinergic effects (Chew et al. 2008). Typically, the entire dose of desipramine or nortriptyline can be given at bedtime.

The tertiary-amine TCAs—amitriptyline, clomipramine, doxepin, and imipramine—can cause significant orthostatic hypotension and anticholinergic effects, including cognitive impairment, and they should be avoided in the elderly (Beers 1997). **(p. 460)**

26.11 Of the atypical antipsychotics currently available in the United States, which has the most published geriatric data for a variety of conditions?

    A. Aripiprazole.
    B. Olanzapine.
    C. Quetiapine.
    D. Risperidone.
    E. Ziprasidone.

The correct response is option D.

Of the typical antipsychotics currently available in the United States, risperidone has the most published geriatric data for a variety of conditions (Alexopoulos et al. 2004; Schneider et al. 2005, 2006a; Sink et al. 2005). Its efficacy and safety in the treatment of behavioral and psychological symptoms of dementia have been demonstrated in several randomized, placebo-controlled trials (e.g., Brodaty et al. 2003; De Deyn et al. 1999, 2005; Katz et al. 1999; Schneider et al. 2006a, 2006b; Sink et al. 2005); randomized comparisons with haloperidol (Chan et al. 2001; De Deyn et al. 1999; Suh et al. 2004), promazine and olanzapine (Gareri et al. 2004), and olanzapine (Fontaine et al. 2003; Mulsant et al. 2004); and uncontrolled studies or large case series (e.g., Herrmann et al. 1998; Irizarry et al. 1999; Lane et al. 2002; Lavretsky and Sultzer 1998; Rainer et al. 2001; Zarate et al. 1997). **(p. 462)**

26.12 On review of all evidence available in 2004, a consensus conference concluded that among the atypical antipsychotics, which of the following had the highest risk for diabetes, weight gain, and dyslipidemia?

 A. Aripiprazole.
 B. Olanzapine.
 C. Quetiapine.
 D. Risperidone.
 E. Ziprasidone.

The correct response is option B.

On review of all evidence available in 2004, a consensus conference concluded that among the atypical antipsychotics, clozapine and olanzapine are associated with the highest risk for diabetes and cause the greatest weight gain and dyslipidemia (American Diabetes Association et al. 2004). **(p. 464)**

26.13 Data suggest that which of the following antipsychotic agents should be first-line for the treatment of psychosis in patients with Parkinson's disease or dementia with Lewy bodies?

 A. Aripiprazole.
 B. Olanzapine.
 C. Quetiapine.
 D. Risperidone.
 E. Ziprasidone.

The correct response is option C.

The good tolerability of quetiapine observed clinically in patients at high risk for extrapyramidal symptoms suggests that quetiapine should be the first-line antipsychotic for older patients with Parkinson's disease, dementia with Lewy bodies, or tardive dyskinesia (Alexopoulos et al. 2004; Poewe 2005). Indeed, the use of quetiapine in late life in patients with Parkinson's disease and drug-induced psychosis has been encouraged (Fernandez et al. 1999, 2002; Menza et al. 1999; Targum and Abbott 2000). **(pp. 464–465)**

26.14 Which of the following side effects has been reported with valproate in as many as half of elderly patients?

 A. Hand tremors.
 B. Pancreatitis.
 C. Elevation in liver enzymes.
 D. Thrombocytopenia.
 E. Transient elevations in blood ammonia levels.

The correct response is option D.

Thrombocytopenia can occur in as many as half of elderly patients treated with valproate and may ensue at lower total drug levels than in younger patients (Conley et al. 2001).

Sedation, nausea, weight gain, and hand tremors are common dose-related side effects. Mild stomach upset may be decreased by use of the enteric-coated divalproex salt. Also dose related are reversible elevations in liver enzymes and transient elevations in blood ammonia levels (Davis et al. 1994). Liver failure and pancreatitis are rare. Valproate has other metabolic effects of concern to aging patients, such as increases in bone turnover and reductions of serum folate, with concomitant elevations in plasma homocysteine concentrations (Sato et al. 2001; Schwaninger et al. 1999). **(p. 467)**

26.15 Which of the following mood stabilizers is **not** associated with weight gain?

    A. Valproate.
    B. Lamotrigine.
    C. Lithium.
    D. Carbamazepine.
    E. Oxcarbazepine.

The correct response is option B.

In contrast with many other mood stabilizers and antidepressants, lamotrigine does not seem to be associated with weight gain (Morrell et al. 2003). In geriatric patients, rashes were the most common reason for study withdrawal, but they were less frequent with lamotrigine (3%) than with carbamazepine (19%) (Brodie et al. 1999). **(p. 468)**

26.16 If a benzodiazepine must be prescribed to an elderly person for treatment of sleep disturbance, which of the following is preferred?

    A. Clonazepam.
    B. Alprazolam.
    C. Triazolam.
    D. Oxazepam.
    E. Lorazepam.

The correct response is option E.

Lorazepam is preferred for inducing sleep because oxazepam has a relatively slow and erratic absorption. Lorazepam is available in appropriately small doses (0.5-mg pills) and is well absorbed intramuscularly.

In the elderly, compounds with long half-lives (clonazepam, diazepam, and flurazepam) should be avoided. Also, several drugs with shorter half-lives (i.e., alprazolam, triazolam, midazolam, and the nonbenzodiazepines eszopiclone, zaleplon, and zolpidem) undergo phase I hepatic metabolism by cytochrome P450 3A4 that is subject to specific interactions and age-associated decline (Freudenreich and Menza 2000; Greenblatt et al. 1991). Sedatives with very short half-lives may also increase the likelihood that confused elders will awake in the middle of the night to stagger off to the bathroom. Oxazepam and lorazepam do not undergo phase I hepatic metabolism, have no active metabolites, have acceptable half-lives that do not increase with age, and are not subject to drug interactions. **(pp. 468–469)**

TABLE 26–3. Cholinesterase inhibitors

	Clearance	Dosing	Significant side effects	Pharmacodynamics
Donepezil	Half-life = 70–80 hr CYP3A4, 2D6	5–10 mg/day in one dose per day; start at 5 mg at bedtime	Mild nausea, diarrhea, agitation	Reversible acetylcholinesterase inhibition
Galantamine Galantamine ER	Half-life = 7 hr CYP2D6, 3A4	8–24 mg/day divided into two doses; start at 8 mg/ day twice daily	Moderate nausea, vomiting, diarrhea, anorexia, tremor, insomnia	Reversible acetylcholinesterase inhibition; nicotinic modulation may increase acetylcholine release
Rivastigmine	Half-life = 1.25 hr Renal	6–12 mg/day divided into two doses; start at 1.5 mg twice daily, retitrate if drug is stopped	Severe nausea, vomiting, anorexia, weight loss, sweating, dizziness	Pseudoirreversible acetylcholinesterase inhibition, also butylcholinesterase inhibition

Note. ER=extended release.

26.17 Which of the following approved drugs for the treatment of Alzheimer's disease is an uncompetitive antagonist with moderate affinity for *N*-methyl-D-aspartate (NMDA) receptors?

A. Donepezil.
B. Memantine.
C. Rivastigmine.
D. Galantamine.
E. Tacrine.

The correct response is option B.

Memantine, the first drug of this class, is FDA-approved for the treatment of moderate to severe Alzheimer's disease. Glutamatergic overstimulation may cause excitotoxic neuronal damage. As an uncompetitive antagonist with moderate affinity for NMDA receptors, memantine may attenuate neurotoxicity without interfering with glutamate's normal physiological actions.

Four of the five currently approved drugs for Alzheimer's disease in the United States—donepezil, galantamine, rivastigmine, and tacrine—are cholinesterase inhibitors (Table 26–3). The use of tacrine is no longer recommended, however, because of its potential hepatotoxic effects. **(pp. 469–470)**

References

Alexopoulos GS, Katz IR, Reynolds CF 3rd, et al: Pharmacotherapy of depression in older patients: a summary of the expert consensus guidelines. J Psychiatr Pract 7:361–376, 2001

Alexopoulos GS, Streim J, Carpenter D, et al: Using antipsychotic agents in older patients. J Clin Psychiatry 65 (suppl 2):5–104, 2004

American Diabetes Association, American Psychiatric Association, American Association of Clinical Endocrinologists, et al: Consensus development conference on antipsychotic drugs and obesity and diabetes. Diabetes Care 27:596–601, 2004

Aragona M, Inghilleri M: Increased ocular pressure in two patients with narrow angle glaucoma treated with venlafaxine. Clin Neuropharmacol 21:130–131, 1998

Bailer U, Fischer P, Kufferle B, et al: Occurrence of mirtazapine-induced delirium in organic brain disorder. Int Clin Psychopharmacol 15:239–243, 2000

Beers MH: Explicit criteria for determining potentially inappropriate medication use by the elderly. Arch Intern Med 157:1531–1536, 1997

Benazzi F: Urinary retention with venlafaxine-haloperidol combination. Pharmacopsychiatry 30:27, 1997

Brodaty H, Ames D, Snowdon J, et al: A randomized placebo-controlled trial of risperidone for the treatment of aggression, agitation, and psychosis of dementia. J Clin Psychiatry 64:134–143, 2003

Brodie MJ, Overstall PW, Giorgi L: Multicentre, double-blind, randomised comparison between lamotrigine and carbamazepine in elderly patients with newly diagnosed epilepsy. The UK Lamotrigine Elderly Study Group. Epilepsy Res 37:81–87, 1999

Burrows AB, Salzman C, Satlin A, et al: A randomized, placebo-controlled trial of paroxetine in nursing home residents with non-major depression. Depress Anxiety 15:102–110, 2002

Carvajal García-Pando A, García del Pozo J, Sánchez AS, et al: Hepatotoxicity associated with the new antidepressants. J Clin Psychiatry 63:135–137, 2002

Chalon SA, Granier LA, Vandenhende FR, et al: Duloxetine increases serotonin and norepinephrine availability in healthy subjects: a double-blind, controlled study. Neuropsychopharmacology 28:1685–1693, 2003

Chan WC, Lam LC, Choy CN, et al: A double-blind randomised comparison of risperidone and haloperidol in the treatment of behavioural and psychological symptoms in Chinese dementia patients. Int J Geriatr Psychiatry 16:1156–1162, 2001

Chen P, Kales HC, Weintraub D, et al: Antidepressant treatment of veterans with Parkinson's disease and depression: analysis of a national sample. J Geriatr Psychiatry Neurol 20:161–165, 2007

Chew ML, Mulsant BH, Pollock BG, et al: Anticholinergic activity of 107 medications commonly used by older adults. J Am Geriatr Soc 56:1333–1341, 2008

Conley EL, Coley KC, Pollock BG, et al: Prevalence and risk of thrombocytopenia with valproic acid: experience at a psychiatric teaching hospital. Pharmacotherapy 21:1325–1330, 2001

Dalton SO, Sorensen HT, Johansen C: SSRIs and upper gastrointestinal bleeding: what is known and how should it influence prescribing? CNS Drugs 20:143–151, 2006

Davidson J, Watkins L, Owens M, et al: Effects of paroxetine and venlafaxine XR on heart rate variability in depression. J Clin Psychopharmacol 25:480–484, 2005

Davis R, Peters DH, McTavish D: Valproic acid: a reappraisal of its pharmacological properties and clinical efficacy in epilepsy. Drugs 47:332–372, 1994

De Deyn PP, Rabheru K, Rasmussen A, et al: A randomized trial of risperidone, placebo, and haloperidol for behavioral symptoms of dementia. Neurology 53:946–955, 1999

De Deyn PP, Katz IR, Brodaty H, et al: Management of agitation, aggression, and psychosis associated with dementia: a pooled analysis including three randomized, placebo-controlled double-blind trials in nursing home residents treated with risperidone. Clin Neurol Neurosurg 107:497–508, 2005

Doraiswamy PM, Krishnan KR, Oxman T, et al: Does antidepressant therapy improve cognition in elderly depressed patients? J Gerontol A Biol Sci Med Sci 58:M1137–M1144, 2003

Dunner DL, Zisook S, Billow AA, et al: A prospective safety surveillance study for bupropion sustained-release in the treatment of depression. J Clin Psychiatry 59:366–373, 1998

Fernandez HH, Friedman JH, Jacques C, et al: Quetiapine for the treatment of drug-induced psychosis in Parkinson's disease. Mov Disord 14:484–487, 1999

Fernandez HH, Trieschmann ME, Burke MA, et al: Quetiapine for psychosis in Parkinson's disease versus dementia with Lewy bodies. J Clin Psychiatry 63:513–515, 2002

Fontaine CS, Hynan LS, Koch K, et al: A double-blind comparison of olanzapine versus risperidone in the acute treatment of dementia-related behavioral disturbances in extended care facilities. J Clin Psychiatry 64:726–730, 2003

Freudenreich O, Menza M: Zolpidem-related delirium: a case report. J Clin Psychiatry 61:449–450, 2000

Furlan PM, Kallan MJ, Ten Have T, et al: Cognitive and psychomotor effects of paroxetine and sertraline on healthy elderly volunteers. Am J Geriatr Psychiatry 9:429–438, 2001

Gareri P, Cotroneo A, Lacava R, et al: Comparison of the efficacy of new and conventional antipsychotic drugs in the treatment of behavioral and psychological symptoms of dementia (BPSD). Arch Gerontol Geriatr Suppl 9:207–215, 2004

Goldstein DJ, Lu Y, Detke MJ, et al: Duloxetine vs placebo in patients with painful diabetic neuropathy. Pain 116:109–118, 2005

Greenblatt DJ, Harmatz JS, Shapiro L, et al: Sensitivity to triazolam in the elderly. N Engl J Med 324:1691–1698, 1991

Herrmann N, Rivard MF, Flynn M, et al: Risperidone for the treatment of behavioral disturbances in dementia: a case series. J Neuropsychiatry Clin Neurosci 10:220–223, 1998

Howard WT, Warnock JK: Bupropion-induced psychosis. Am J Psychiatry 156:2017–2018, 1999

Hudson JI, Wohlreich MM, Kajdasz DK, et al: Safety and tolerability of duloxetine in the treatment of major depressive disorder: analysis of pooled data from eight placebo-controlled clinical trials. Hum Psychopharmacol 20:327–341, 2005

Hutchison LC: Mirtazapine and bone marrow suppression: a case report. J Am Geriatr Soc 49:1129–1130, 2001

Irizarry MC, Ghaemi SN, Lee-Cherry ER, et al: Risperidone treatment of behavioral disturbances in outpatients with dementia. J Neuropsychiatry Clin Neurosci 11:336–342, 1999

Johnson EM, Whyte E, Mulsant BH, et al: Cardiovascular changes associated with venlafaxine in the treatment of late life depression. Am J Geriatr Psychiatry 14:796–802, 2006

Katz IR, Jeste DV, Mintzer JE, et al: Comparison of risperidone and placebo for psychosis and behavioral disturbances associated with dementia: a randomized, double-blind trial. Risperidone Study Group. J Clin Psychiatry 60:107–115, 1999

Kiev A, Masco HL, Wenger TL, et al: The cardiovascular effects of bupropion and nortriptyline in depressed outpatients. Ann Clin Psychiatry 6:107–115, 1994

Kirwin JL, Goren JL: Duloxetine: a dual serotonin-norepinephrine reuptake inhibitor for treatment of major depressive disorder. Pharmacotherapy 25:396–410, 2005

Kroenke K, West SL, Swindle R, et al: Similar effectiveness of paroxetine, fluoxetine, and sertraline in primary care: a randomized trial. JAMA 286:2947–2955, 2001

Lane HY, Chang YC, Su MH, et al: Shifting from haloperidol to risperidone for behavioral disturbances in dementia: safety, response predictors, and mood effects. J Clin Psychopharmacol 22:4–10, 2002

Lavretsky H, Sultzer D: A structured trial of risperidone for the treatment of agitation in dementia. Am J Geriatr Psychiatry 6:127–135, 1998

Lessard E, Yessine MA, Hamelin BA, et al: Influence of CYP2D6 activity on the disposition and cardiovascular toxicity of the antidepressant agent venlafaxine in humans. Pharmacogenetics 9:435–443, 1999

Liu B, Anderson G, Mittmann N, et al: Use of selective serotonin reuptake inhibitors or tricyclic antidepressants and risk of hip fractures in elderly people. Lancet 351:1303–1307, 1998

Looper KJ: Potential medical and surgical complications of serotonergic antidepressants. Psychosomatics 48:1–9, 2007

Lucena MI, Andrade RJ, Gomez-Outes A, et al: Acute liver failure after treatment with nefazodone. Dig Dis Sci 44:2577–2579, 1999

Mamo DC, Sweet RA, Mulsant BH, et al: Effect of nortriptyline and paroxetine on extrapyramidal signs and symptoms: a prospective double-blind study in depressed elderly patients. Am J Geriatr Psychiatry 8:226–231, 2000

Mariappan P, Ballantyne Z, N'Dow JMO, et al: Serotonin and noradrenaline reuptake inhibitors (SNRI) for stress urinary incontinence in adults. Cochrane Database Syst Rev (3):CD004742, 2005

Menza MM, Palermo B, Mark M: Quetiapine as an alternative to clozapine in the treatment of dopamimetic psychosis in patients with Parkinson's disease. Ann Clin Psychiatry 11:141–144, 1999

Morrell MJ, Isojärvi J, Taylor AE, et al: Higher androgens and weight gain with valproate compared with lamotrigine for epilepsy. Epilepsy Res 54:189–199, 2003

Mulsant BH, Alexopoulos GS, Reynolds CF 3rd, et al: Pharmacological treatment of depression in older primary care patients: the PROSPECT algorithm. Int J Geriatr Psychiatry 16:585–592, 2001

Mulsant BH, Gharabawi GM, Bossie CA, et al: Correlates of anticholinergic activity in patients with dementia and psychosis treated with risperidone or olanzapine. J Clin Psychiatry 65:1708–1714, 2004

National Collaborating Centre for Mental Health: Management of Depression in Primary and Secondary Care (Clinical Guideline 23). London, England, National Institute for Clinical Excellence, 2004

Nelson JC, Wohlreich MM, Mallinckrodt CH, et al: Duloxetine for the treatment of major depressive disorder in older patients. Am J Geriatr Psychiatry 13:227–235, 2005

Newhouse PA, Krishnan KR, Doraiswamy PM, et al: A double-blind comparison of sertraline and fluoxetine in depressed elderly outpatients. J Clin Psychiatry 61:559–568, 2000

Nicholas LM, Ford AL, Esposito SM, et al: The effects of mirtazapine on plasma lipid profiles in healthy subjects. J Clin Psychiatry 64:883–889, 2003

Nyth AL, Gottfries CG: The clinical efficacy of citalopram in treatment of emotional disturbances in dementia disorders: a Nordic multicentre study. Br J Psychiatry 157:894–901, 1990

Nyth AL, Gottfries CG, Lyby K, et al: A controlled multicenter clinical study of citalopram and placebo in elderly depressed patients with and without concomitant dementia. Acta Psychiatr Scand 86:138–145, 1992

Oslin DW, Ten Have TR, Streim JE, et al: Probing the safety of medications in the frail elderly: evidence from a randomized clinical trial of sertraline and venlafaxine in depressed nursing home residents. J Clin Psychiatry 64:875–882, 2003

Poewe W: Treatment of dementia with Lewy bodies and Parkinson's disease dementia. Mov Disord 20 (suppl 12):S77–S82, 2005

Pollock BG, Laghrissi-Thode F, Wagner WR: Evaluation of platelet activation in depressed patients with ischemic heart disease after paroxetine or nortriptyline treatment. J Clin Psychopharmacol 20:137–140, 2000

Rabins PV, Lyketsos CG: Antipsychotic drugs in dementia: what should be made of the risks? JAMA 294:1963–1965, 2005

Rainer MK, Masching AJ, Ertl MG, et al: Effect of risperidone on behavioral and psychological symptoms and cognitive function in dementia. J Clin Psychiatry 62:894–900, 2001

Raji MA, Brady SR: Mirtazapine for treatment of depression and comorbidities in Alzheimer disease. Ann Pharmacother 35:1024–1027, 2001

Raskin J, Wiltse CG, Siegal A, et al: Efficacy of duloxetine on cognition, depression, and pain in elderly patients with major depressive disorder: an 8-week, double-blind, placebo-controlled trial. Am J Psychiatry 164:900–909, 2007

Reznik I, Rosen Y, Rosen B: An acute ischaemic event associated with the use of venlafaxine: a case report and proposed pathophysiological mechanisms. J Psychopharmacol 13:193–195, 1999

Richards JB, Papaioannou A, Adachi JD for the Canadian Multicentre Osteoporosis Study Research Group: Effect of selective serotonin reuptake inhibitors on the risk of fracture. Arch Intern Med 167:188–194, 2007

Ridout F, Meadows R, Johnsen S, et al: A placebo controlled investigation into the effects of paroxetine and mirtazapine on measures related to car driving performance. Hum Psychopharmacol 18:261–269, 2003

Roose SP, Dalack GW, Glassman AH, et al: Cardiovascular effects of bupropion in depressed patients with heart disease. Am J Psychiatry 148:512–516, 1991

Roose SP, Nelson JC, Salzman C, et al: Mirtazapine in the Nursing Home Study Group: open-label study of mirtazapine orally disintegrating tablets in depressed patients in the nursing home. Curr Med Res Opin 19:737–746, 2003

Saiz-Ruiz J, Ibanez A, Diaz-Marsa M, et al: Nefazodone in the treatment of elderly patients with depressive disorders: a prospective, observational study. CNS Drugs 16:635–643, 2002

Sato Y, Kondo I, Ishida S, et al: Decreased bone mass and increased bone turnover with valproate therapy in adults with epilepsy. Neurology 57:445–449, 2001

Schneider LS, Olin JT: Efficacy of acute treatment for geriatric depression. Int Psychogeriatr 7(suppl):7–25, 1995

Schneider LS, Dagerman KS, Insel P: Risk of death with atypical antipsychotic drug treatment for dementia: meta-analysis of randomized placebo-controlled trials. JAMA 294:1934–1943, 2005

Schneider LS, Dagerman KS, Insel PS: Efficacy and adverse effects of atypical antipsychotics for dementia: meta-analysis of randomized placebo-controlled trials. Am J Geriatr Psychiatry 14:191–210, 2006a

Schneider LS, Tariot PN, Dagerman KS, et al: Effectiveness of atypical antipsychotic drugs in patients with Alzheimer's disease. N Engl J Med 355:1525–1538, 2006b

Schwaninger M, Ringleb P, Winter R, et al: Elevated plasma concentrations of homocysteine in antiepileptic drug treatment. Epilepsia 40:345–350, 1999

Semenchuk MR, Sherman S, Davis B: Double-blind, randomized trial of bupropion SR for the treatment of neuropathic pain. Neurology 57:1583–1588, 2001

Sink KM, Holden KF, Yaffe K: Pharmacological treatment of neuropsychiatric symptoms of dementia: a review of the evidence. JAMA 293:596–608, 2005

Solai LK, Mulsant BH, Pollock BG: Selective serotonin reuptake inhibitors for late-life depression: a comparative review. Drugs Aging 18:355–368, 2001

Stimmel GL, Dopheide JA, Stahl SM: Mirtazapine: an antidepressant with noradrenergic and specific serotonergic effects. Pharmacotherapy 17:10–21, 1997

Suh GH, Son HG, Ju YS, et al: A randomized, double-blind, crossover comparison of risperidone and haloperidol in Korean dementia patients with behavioral disturbances. Am J Geriatr Psychiatry 12:509–516, 2004

Targum SD, Abbott JL: Efficacy of quetiapine in Parkinson's patients with psychosis. J Clin Psychopharmacol 20:54–60, 2000

Tashkin D, Kanner R, Bailey W, et al: Smoking cessation in patients with chronic obstructive pulmonary disease: a double-blind, placebo-controlled, randomised trial. Lancet 357:1571–1575, 2001

Thase ME: Effects of venlafaxine on blood pressure: a meta-analysis of original data from 3744 depressed patients. J Clin Psychiatry 59:502–508, 1998

Wingen M, Bothmer J, Langer S, et al: Actual driving performance and psychomotor function in healthy subjects after acute and subchronic treatment with escitalopram, mirtazapine, and placebo: a crossover trial. J Clin Psychiatry 66:436–443, 2005

Zarate CA Jr, Baldessarini RJ, Siegel AJ, et al: Risperidone in the elderly: a pharmacoepidemiologic study. J Clin Psychiatry 58:311–317, 1997

Zimmer B, Kant R, Zeiler D, et al: Antidepressant efficacy and cardiovascular safety of venlafaxine in young vs old patients with comorbid medical disorders. Int J Psychiatry Med 27:353–364, 1997

Chapter 27

Electroconvulsive Therapy

Select the single best response for each question.

27.1 Electroconvulsive therapy (ECT) has been demonstrated to have efficacy in testing a number of specific conditions or disorders. For which of the following has ECT **not** been shown to be efficacious?

   A. Severe nonmelancholic depression.
   B. Negative symptoms of schizophrenia.
   C. Acute mania.
   D. Bipolar depression.
   E. Catatonia.

The correct response is option B.

A disorder for which ECT appears to have efficacy is schizophrenia. Although ECT was first employed as a treatment for this condition, the superior response to ECT of patients with mood disorders was soon evident (Weiner and Krystal 2001). Following the development of antipsychotic medications in the late 1950s, the use of ECT as a treatment for schizophrenia gradually declined. Regardless, a number of studies have suggested that antipsychotic medications and ECT have comparable efficacy (Fink and Sackeim 1996; Krueger and Sackeim 1995). In addition, evidence suggests that for treatment of acute psychotic episodes, the combination of antipsychotic medications and ECT may have greater efficacy than either ECT or medications alone (Klapheke 1993; Sajatovic and Meltzer 1993). However, no evidence indicates that ECT has efficacy for the treatment of deficit or "negative" symptoms of schizophrenia (Weiner and Krystal 2001).

ECT appears to be effective in treating both melancholic and severe nonmelancholic subtypes of depression (Sackeim and Rush 1995), as well as bipolar and unipolar major depression (Weiner and Krystal 2001). In addition, it may be particularly effective in treating psychotic major depression (Petrides et al. 2001; Sobin et al. 1996).

Although ECT is used more frequently for major depression than for other illnesses and the vast majority of ECT research studies have been carried out on this condition, evidence suggests that ECT has efficacy in a number of other mental disorders. In the treatment of acute mania, ECT has been reported to achieve a response rate as high as 80%, to have efficacy equal to that of lithium, and to have a significant advantage over lithium in patients who have not responded to lithium or antipsychotic medication (Mukherjee et al. 1994; Small et al. 1988).

Catatonia, which can be associated with both schizophrenia and mood disorders, is highly responsive to ECT (Krystal and Coffey 1997). **(pp. 486–487)**

27.2 ECT is a highly effective treatment for a number of neuropsychiatric conditions; however, some patients who receive ECT for depression will relapse within 1 year after treatment with ECT, even when treated with typical continuation or maintenance pharmacotherapy. What is the estimated relapse rate for depressed patients 1 year after ECT treatment and when continued on pharmacotherapy?

   A. 5%–10%.
   B. 15%–20%.
   C. 25%–30%.
   D. 40%–49%.
   E. 50%–60%.

The correct response is option E.

Although ECT is a highly effective treatment for a number of neuropsychiatric conditions, it is not a "cure" that ensures future episodes will not occur (Weiner and Krystal 2001; Weiner et al. 2000). Also, evidence indicates that the relapse rate of major depressive disorder may be particularly high for older adults (Huuhka et al. 2004). As a result, it is important to institute some form of continuation or maintenance therapy (American Psychiatric Association 2001). This point is underscored by the findings from a study by Sackeim et al. (2001), in which roughly 80% of patients successfully treated with ECT for major depression relapsed within 6 months. Most commonly, continuation or maintenance pharmacotherapy is instituted after a successful course of ECT. Nevertheless, prophylactic pharmacotherapy is not universally effective, and roughly 50%–60% of depressed patients will relapse within a year of the end of the ECT course when treated with typical continuation or maintenance pharmacotherapy (Sackeim et al. 1990, 2001). **(p. 487)**

27.3 Pharmacotherapy is usually indicated after a successful course of ECT unless one of certain specific conditions exists. All of the following are examples of these contraindicating conditions *except*

   A. The patient has a preference for maintenance ECT.
   B. Maintenance pharmacotherapy has failed in the past.
   C. The patient is intolerant of medications.
   D. The patient has previously responded to maintenance ECT.
   E. The patient has a medical illness that precludes medication.

The correct response is option D.

At the present time, pharmacotherapy is usually instituted after a successful course of ECT unless at least one of the following conditions exists: 1) prophylactic pharmacotherapy has failed in the past, 2) patient is intolerant of medications, 3) patient has a medical illness that contraindicates medication management, or 4) patient has a preference for prophylactic ECT (American Psychiatric Association 2001; Weiner and Krystal 2001). **(p. 487)**

27.4 Objective and subjective memory side effects of ECT have been shown to be greater in degree and duration under which of the following conditions?

   A. Lower stimulus intensity.
   B. More time between treatments.
   C. Larger number of ECT treatments.
   D. Unilateral placement of electrodes.
   E. Lower dosages of barbiturate anesthetic.

The correct response is option C.

Both the degree and the duration of objective and subjective memory side effects of ECT vary substantially among individuals who receive ECT. A number of research studies have identified factors that can affect objective memory side effects of ECT (American Psychiatric Association 2001). Compared with unilateral placement of stimulus electrodes, bilateral placement has repeatedly been shown to increase the risk of amnesia (Stoppe et al. 2006). In addition, greater risk is associated with higher stimulus intensity (compared with the seizure threshold), larger numbers of ECT treatments, higher dosages of barbiturate anesthetic, and less time between treatments. Furthermore, some patients—including those taking lithium and medications with anticholinergic properties, as well as those with preexisting cerebral disease—appear to be at increased risk of cognitive side effects (American Psychiatric Association 2001). Individuals with diseases affecting the basal ganglia and subcortical white matter may be at particular risk (Figiel et al. 1990) **(pp. 488–489).**

27.5 Certain psychotropic medications should be avoided or maintained at the lowest possible levels during ECT treatment. Which of the following is one of these medications?

A. Lithium.
B. Haloperidol.
C. Sertraline.
D. Olanzapine.
E. Desipramine.

The correct response is option A.

When possible, antidepressant medications should be chosen that have relatively fewer effects on cardiac function. The following psychotropic medications are among those that are best avoided or maintained at the lowest possible levels: 1) lithium—it may increase the risks for delirium or prolonged seizures; 2) benzodiazepines—their anticonvulsant properties may decrease efficacy (but can be reversed with flumazenil at the time of ECT) (Krystal et al. 1998); 3) antiepileptic drugs—their anticonvulsant properties may decrease efficacy, but such drugs may be needed in those with epilepsy or with very brittle bipolar disorder (in which case they should be withheld the night before and the morning of treatment if possible); 4) bupropion and clozapine—they may increase the risk of prolonged seizures (the dosage should be kept at low to moderate levels). **(pp. 493–494)**

References

American Psychiatric Association: The Practice of ECT: Recommendations for Treatment, Training, and Privileging. Washington, DC, American Psychiatric Press, 2001

Figiel GS, Coffey CE, Djang WT, et al: Brain magnetic resonance imaging findings in ECT-induced delirium. J Neuropsychiatry Clin Neurosci 2:53–58, 1990

Fink M, Sackeim HA: Convulsive therapy in schizophrenia? Schizophr Bull 22:27–39, 1996

Huuhka M, Korpisammal L, Haataja R, et al: One-year outcome of elderly inpatients with major depressive disorder treated with ECT and antidepressants. J ECT 20:179–185, 2004

Klapheke MM: Combining ECT and antipsychotic agents: benefits and risks. Convuls Ther 9:241–255, 1993

Krueger RB, Sackeim HA: Electroconvulsive therapy and schizophrenia, in Schizophrenia. Edited by Hirsch SR, Weinberger D. Oxford, UK, Blackwell, 1995, pp 503–545

Krystal AD, Coffey CE: Neuropsychiatric considerations in the use of electroconvulsive therapy. J Neuropsychiatry Clin Neurosci 9:283–292, 1997

Krystal AD, Watts BV, Weiner RD, et al: The use of flumazenil in the anxious and benzodiazepine-dependent ECT patient. J ECT 14:5–14, 1998

Mukherjee S, Sackeim HA, Schnur DB: Electroconvulsive therapy of acute mania episodes: a review of 50 years' experience. Am J Psychiatry 151:169–176, 1994

Petrides G, Fink M, Husain MM, et al: ECT remission rates in psychotic versus nonpsychotic depressed patients: a report from CORE. J ECT 17:244–253, 2001

Sackeim HA, Rush AJ: Melancholia and response to ECT. Am J Psychiatry 152:1242–1243, 1995

Sackeim HA, Prudic J, Devanand DP, et al: The impact of medication resistance and continuation pharmacotherapy on relapse following response to electroconvulsive therapy in major depression. J Clin Psychopharmacol 10:96–104, 1990

Sackeim HA, Haskett RF, Mulsant BH, et al: Continuation pharmacotherapy in the prevention of relapse following electroconvulsive therapy: a randomized controlled trial. JAMA 285:1299–1307, 2001

Sajatovic M, Meltzer HY: The effect of short-term electroconvulsive treatment plus neuroleptics in treatment-resistant schizophrenia and schizoaffective disorder. Convuls Ther 9:167–173, 1993

Small JG, Klapper MH, Kellams JJ, et al: Electroconvulsive treatment compared with lithium in the management of manic states. Arch Gen Psychiatry 45:727–732, 1988

Sobin C, Prudic J, Devanand DP, et al: Who responds to electroconvulsive therapy? A comparison of effective and ineffective forms of treatment. Br J Psychiatry 169:322–328, 1996

Stoppe A, Louza M, Rosa M, et al: Fixed high-dose electroconvulsive therapy in the elderly with depression: a double-blind, randomized comparison of efficacy and tolerability between unilateral and bilateral electrode placement. J ECT 22:92–99, 2006

Weiner RD, Krystal AD: Electroconvulsive therapy, in Treatments of Psychiatric Disorders, 3rd Edition. Edited by Gabbard GO, Rush AJ. Washington, DC, American Psychiatric Press, 2001, pp 1267–1293

Weiner RD, Coffey CE, Krystal AD: Electroconvulsive therapy in the medical and neurologic patient, in Psychiatric Care of the Medical Patient, 2nd Edition. Edited by Stoudemire A, Fogel BS, Greenberg D. New York, Oxford University Press, 2000, pp 419–428

Chapter 28

Nutrition and Physical Activity

Select the single best response for each question.

28.1 Adherence to the Mediterranean diet has been associated with a reduced risk for cognitive decline. Which of the following is a component of the Mediterranean diet?

    A. High intake of trans-unsaturated fats.
    B. No ethanol consumption.
    C. High intake of saturated fats.
    D. High intake of poly-unsaturated fats.
    E. Low intake of mono-unsaturated fats.

The correct response is option D.

The type of fat may be an important determinant of cognitive health. Dietary fats are divided into four general categories: saturated, trans-unsaturated, mono-unsaturated, and poly-unsaturated, with the latter subdivided into omega-6 and omega-3 fats. Saturated and trans-unsaturated fats are likely detrimental to cognitive as well as overall health, whereas mono-unsaturated and poly-unsaturated (especially omega-3) fats are associated with a reduced risk of cognitive decline and dementia (Solfrizzi et al. 2006). Adherence to the Mediterranean diet, characterized by high intake of mono-unsaturated and omega-3 fats, moderate ethanol consumption, and low intake of saturated fats, has been associated with a reduced risk for cognitive decline (Scarmeas et al. 2006). **(p. 503)**

28.2 There are three major components of nutritional assessment: dietary, biochemical, and clinical. The most commonly used biochemical assessment is for one or more markers of protein status. Which of the following markers has a very short half-life of 2–4 hours and a relatively small body pool, making it very sensitive to nutritional changes?

    A. Albumin.
    B. Prealbumin.
    C. Insulin-like growth factor 1 (IGF-1).
    D. Insulin.
    E. Transthyretin.

The correct response is option C.

The most commonly used biochemical assessment is for one or more markers of protein status. Albumin is one of the most abundant and commonly measured serum proteins. However, albumin has a relatively long half-life (18 days), and levels also are known to decrease with age. Because chronic or acute inflammation, advanced liver disease, heart failure, nephrotic syndrome, and protein-losing enteropathy can all result in hypoalbuminemia, serum albumin is not recommended as a sole marker of nutritional status (Sullivan et al. 2002). Other serum proteins that have been studied as protein status markers are prealbumin (or transthyretin) and IGF-1. Prealbumin is a transport protein for thyroxine with a half-life of 2 days. Prealbumin levels usually show daily improvements with good nutritional repletion. IGF-1 is a peptide produced by the liver, for which levels drop rapidly during starvation and increase during nutritional repletion. IGF-1 has a very short half-life of 2–4 hours and a relatively small body pool, making it very sensitive to nutritional changes. In hospitalized older adults, low IGF-1 levels are associated with higher morbidity and life-threatening complications (Sullivan and Carter 1994). (p. 509)

28.3 Although most nutritional experts recommend that all older adults take a multivitamin/mineral supplement, specific nutrients have been associated with adverse outcomes. Excessive intake of which of the following nutrients can interfere with copper status and impair immune function?

    A. Vitamin A.
    B. Zinc.
    C. Vitamin E.
    D. Folic acid.
    E. Iron.

The correct response is option B.

Although most experts support the recommendation that all older adults take a multivitamin/mineral supplement, it is important to consider carefully the types and amounts of supplements being chosen. Potential risks from excessive intakes of specific nutrients include the possibility of increased risk of hip fractures with vitamin A (Feskanich et al. 2002; Melhus et al. 1998) and the aggravation of iron overload by mineral supplements containing iron. Supplemental iron, unless given to remedy an anemic condition, may be unwise for those who are homozygous or heterozygous for mutations of the hemochromatosis-associated gene, because even relatively modest amounts of supplemental iron could increase the likelihood of diabetes and cardiovascular disease in these individuals (Garry et al. 1982). A recent meta-analysis linked use of high-dose vitamin E supplements with an increase in all-cause mortality (Miller et al. 2005). Long-term zinc supplementation, especially at higher doses, can interfere with copper status and impair immune function (Bogden 2004; McClain et al. 2002). Of particular concern in regard to nutrition and mental health is the possibility that large intakes of folate (or folic acid) could mask symptoms of a vitamin B_{12} deficiency. The interaction of folate and vitamin B_{12} with metabolism makes it essential to ensure that intake and status of these two nutrients are in balance. **(p. 513)**

28.4 A panel composed of public health, behavioral science, epidemiology, exercise science, medicine, and gerontology experts released recommendations on physical activity in older adults. Which of the following were its recommendations for aerobic activities?

    A. Mild-intensity aerobic activity at least 10 minutes each day, 7 days a week.
    B. Moderate-intensity aerobic activity at least 10 minutes each day, 7 days a week.
    C. Moderate-intensity aerobic activity at least 20 minutes each day, 7 days a week.
    D. Moderate-intensity aerobic activity at least 30 minutes each day, 5 days a week.
    E. Maximal-intensity aerobic activity at least 30 minutes each day, 7 days a week.

The correct response is option D.

A panel composed of public health, behavioral science, epidemiology, exercise science, medicine, and gerontology experts has released recommendations on physical activity of older adults based on prior recommendations from the American College of Sports Medicine and the American Heart Association for adults as well as relevant evidence from primary research and existing consensus statements (Nelson et al. 2007).

    Moderate-intensity activity beyond routine activities of daily living and more than 10 minutes in duration is necessary to benefit the health of older adults. Moderate-intensity aerobic activity is best described as producing noticeable increases in heart rate and breathing and ranking on a level of 5 or 6 on a 10-point scale, in which sitting is 0 and maximal effort is 10. To promote and maintain health, older adults should participate in such aerobic activity for at least 30 minutes, 5 days each week. **(p. 514)**

28.5   A number of nutrients have been linked to depression. Cross-sectional studies have associated depression with low levels of one of the nutrients below; however, longitudinal studies have failed to find an association. Which nutrient do these findings refer to?

   A. Pyridoxine (B_6).
   B. Folate (B_9).
   C. Cobalamin (B_{12}).
   D. Omega-3 fatty acids.
   E. Saturated fats.

The correct response is option C.

A number of nutrients have been specifically linked to depression, including the B vitamins and omega-3 fatty acids. Of the B vitamins, pyridoxine (B_6), cobalamin (B_{12}), and folate (B_9) are essential for serotonin production and myelin formation and have been implicated in depression. Pyridoxine deficiency is common in the elderly, and low levels of pyridoxine have been correlated with depression (Bell et al. 1991; Stewart et al. 1984; Tolonen et al. 1988). However, studies of these factors have not demonstrated that low pyridoxine levels or pyridoxine deficiency cause depression.

Cobalamin deficiency is also common in the elderly and is mostly attributable to insufficient intrinsic factor, which is necessary for gastrointestinal absorption of B_{12} (Andres et al. 2004). Although prolonged B_{12} deficiency has been shown to cause irreversible neurological damage, its relationship to depression is less clear. Although cross-sectional population studies have associated depression with low B_{12} (Penninx et al. 2000; Tiemeier et al. 2002), longitudinal studies have failed to find an association between depression and B_{12} (Eussen et al. 2002; Sachdev et al. 2005).

Folate has been studied extensively in relationship to depression, and its importance may relate to neuronal (serotonin or myelin production) or vascular (including homocysteine metabolism) functions. Clinical studies have found folate levels to be inversely associated with both depression and depression severity (Abou-Saleh and Coppen 1986; Bell et al. 1990; Botez et al. 1982; Bottiglieri et al. 1990; Ghadirian et al. 1980; Hunter et al. 1967; Levitt and Joffe 1989). However, many of these studies failed to control for comorbid disease and other risk factors for depression. In addition, the majority of population and community studies have found no association between folate status and depression (Bjelland et al. 2003; Eussen et al. 2002; Lindeman et al. 2000; Penninx et al. 2000).

There is evidence that omega-3 fatty acid metabolism is altered with depression, but dietary studies have been conflicting (Adams et al. 1996; Maes et al. 1999). Population studies have shown that fish consumption may be protective for depression, associating a higher fish consumption with a decreased risk of depression (Hibbeln 1998; Tanskanen et al. 2001). However, a fish and fish oil supplementation trial conducted in the United Kingdom did not confirm a beneficial effect on depression (Ness et al. 2003). **(pp. 504–505)**

References

Abou-Saleh MT, Coppen A: The biology of folate in depression: implications for nutritional hypotheses of the psychoses. J Psychiatr Res 20:91–101, 1986

Adams PB, Lawson S, Sanigorski A, et al: Arachidonic acid to eicosapentaenoic acid ratio in blood correlates positively with clinical symptoms of depression. Lipids 31(suppl):S157–S161, 1996

Andres E, Loukili NH, Noel E, et al: Vitamin B12 (cobalamin) deficiency in elderly patients. CMAJ 171:251–259, 2004

Bell IR, Edman JS, Marby DW, et al: Vitamin B12 and folate status in acute geropsychiatric inpatients: affective and cognitive characteristics of a vitamin nondeficient population. Biol Psychiatry 27:125–137, 1990

Bell IR, Edman JS, Morrow FD, et al: B complex vitamin patterns in geriatric and young adult inpatients with major depression. J Am Geriatr Soc 39:252–257, 1991

Bjelland I, Tell GS, Vollset SE, et al: Folate, vitamin B12, homocysteine, and the MTHFR 677C→T polymorphism in anxiety and depression: the Hordaland Homocysteine Study. Arch Gen Psychiatry 60:618–626, 2003

Bogden JD: Influence of zinc on immunity in the elderly. J Nutr Health Aging 8:48–54, 2004

Botez MI, Young SN, Bachevalier J, et al: Effect of folic acid and vitamin B12 deficiencies on 5-hydroxyindoleacetic acid in human cerebrospinal fluid. Ann Neurol 12:479–484, 1982

Bottiglieri T, Hyland K, Laundy M, et al: Enhancement of recovery from psychiatric illness by methylfolate. Lancet 336:1579–1580, 1990

Eussen SJ, Ferry M, Hininger I, et al: Five year changes in mental health and associations with vitamin B12/folate status of elderly Europeans. J Nutr Health Aging 6:43–50, 2002

Feskanich D, Singh V, Willett WC, et al: Vitamin A intake and hip fractures among postmenopausal women. JAMA 287:47–54, 2002

Garry PJ, Goodwin JS, Hunt WC, et al: Nutritional status in a healthy elderly population: dietary and supplemental intakes. Am J Clin Nutr 36:319–331, 1982

Ghadirian AM, Ananth J, Engelsmann F: Folic acid deficiency and depression. Psychosomatics 21:926–929, 1980

Hibbeln JR: Fish consumption and major depression. Lancet 351:1213, 1998

Hunter R, Jones M, Jones TG, et al: Serum B12 and folate concentrations in mental patients. Br J Psychiatry 113:1291–1295, 1967

Levitt AJ, Joffe RT: Folate, B12, and life course of depressive illness. Biol Psychiatry 25:867–872, 1989

Lindeman RD, Romero LJ, Koehler KM, et al: Serum vitamin B12, C and folate concentrations in the New Mexico elder health survey: correlations with cognitive and affective functions. J Am Coll Nutr 19:68–76, 2000

Maes M, Christophe A, Delanghe J, et al: Lowered omega3 polyunsaturated fatty acids in serum phospholipids and cholesteryl esters of depressed patients. Psychiatry Res 85:275–291, 1999

McClain CJ, McClain M, Barve S, et al: Trace metals and the elderly. Clin Geriatr Med 18:801–818, 2002

Melhus H, Michaelsson K, Kindmark A, et al: Excessive dietary intake of vitamin A is associated with reduced bone mineral density and increased risk for hip fracture. Ann Intern Med 129:770–778, 1998

Miller ER 3rd, Pastor-Barriuso R, Dalal D, et al: Meta-analysis: high-dosage vitamin E supplementation may increase all-cause mortality. Ann Intern Med 142:37–46, 2005

Nelson ME, Rejeski WJ, Blair SN, et al: Physical activity and public health in older adults: recommendation from the American College of Sports Medicine and the American Heart Association. Med Sci Sports Exerc 39:1435–1445, 2007

Ness AR, Gallacher JE, Bennett PD, et al: Advice to eat fish and mood: a randomised controlled trial in men with angina. Nutr Neurosci 6:63–65, 2003

Penninx BW, Guralnik JM, Ferrucci L, et al: Vitamin B(12) deficiency and depression in physically disabled older women: epidemiologic evidence from the Women's Health and Aging Study. Am J Psychiatry 157:715–721, 2000

Sachdev PS, Parslow RA, Lux O, et al: Relationship of homocysteine, folic acid and vitamin B12 with depression in a middle-aged community sample. Psychol Med 35:529–538, 2005

Scarmeas N, Stern Y, Tang MX, et al: Mediterranean diet and risk for Alzheimer's disease. Ann Neurol 59:912–921, 2006

Solfrizzi V, Colacicco AM, D'Introno A, et al: Dietary intake of unsaturated fatty acids and age-related cognitive decline: a 8.5-year follow-up of the Italian Longitudinal Study on Aging. Neurobiol Aging 27:1694–1704, 2006

Stewart JW, Harrison W, Quitkin F, et al: Low B6 levels in depressed outpatients. Biol Psychiatry 19:613–616, 1984

Sullivan DH, Carter WJ: Insulin-like growth factor I as an indicator of protein-energy undernutrition among metabolically stable hospitalized elderly. J Am Coll Nutr 13:184–191, 1994

Sullivan DH, Bopp MM, Roberson PK: Protein-energy undernutrition and life-threatening complications among the hospitalized elderly. J Gen Intern Med 17:923–932, 2002

Tanskanen A, Hibbeln JR, Hintikka J, et al: Fish consumption, depression, and suicidality in a general population. Arch Gen Psychiatry 58:512–513, 2001

Tiemeier H, van Tuijl HR, Hofman A, et al: Vitamin B12, folate, and homocysteine in depression: the Rotterdam Study. Am J Psychiatry 159:2099–2101, 2002

Tolonen M, Schrijver J, Westermarck T, et al: Vitamin B6 status of Finnish elderly. Comparison with Dutch younger adults and elderly. The effect of supplementation. Int J Vitam Nutr Res 58:73–77, 1988

Chapter 29

Individual and Group Psychotherapy

Select the single best response for each question.

29.1 In the first known randomized trial examining cognitive-behavioral therapy (CBT) as a medication augmentation therapy, more than 100 depressed older adults were assigned to three treatment approaches: CBT alone, medication alone, or combined CBT and medication. What were the major findings?

    A. CBT alone had the greatest improvement over 16–20 weeks of treatment.

    B. CBT alone was significantly better than medication alone.

    C. The combined CBT and medication group reported the greatest improvements over 16–20 weeks of treatment.

    D. Medication alone was significantly better than CBT alone.

    E. Medication alone had the greatest improvement over 16–20 weeks of treatment.

The correct response is option C.

In the first known randomized trial examining CBT as a medication augmentation strategy, Thompson et al. (2001) assessed 102 depressed older adults. Patients were assigned to one of three treatment conditions: 1) CBT alone, 2) medication alone, or 3) combined CBT and medication. Although all three groups showed improvements in depressive symptoms over 16–20 weeks of treatment, the combined-therapy group had the greatest improvements. A significant difference was found between the combined-therapy and the medication-only groups. The CBT-alone group showed similar improvements as the combined-therapy group, but the superiority of CBT alone over medication alone did not reach a significant level. This study supports conclusions by Reynolds et al. (1999) that a combined medication plus psychotherapy approach may be optimal for the treatment of depression in older adults. **(p. 523)**

29.2 Which of the following is a manualized treatment focused on four components (grief, interpersonal disputes, role transitions, and interpersonal deficits) that are hypothesized to lead to or maintain depression?

    A. Social problem-solving therapy (PST).

    B. Interpersonal psychotherapy (IPT).

    C. Cognitive-behavioral therapy.

    D. Psychodynamic psychotherapy.

    E. Cognitive therapy.

The correct response is option B.

IPT is a manualized treatment that focuses on four components that are hypothesized to lead to or maintain depression. Whatever its etiology, depression is seen to persist in a social context. The four components of treatment focus are 1) grief (e.g., death of spouse), 2) interpersonal disputes (e.g., conflict with adult children), 3) role transitions (e.g., retirement), and 4) interpersonal deficits (e.g., lack of assertiveness skills). Techniques utilized in treatment include role playing, communication analysis, clarification of the patient's wants and needs, and links between affect and environmental events (Hinrichsen 1997).

PST is based on a model in which ineffective coping under stress is hypothesized to lead to a breakdown of problem-solving abilities and subsequent depression (Nezu 1987; Thompson and Gallagher 1984). Patients are taught a structured format for solving problems that considers problem details, present goals, multiple solutions, specific solution advantages, and assessing the final solution in context. PST ideally refines and augments patients' present strategies to improve their ability to handle day-to-day problems.

Psychodynamic psychotherapy is based on psychoanalytic theory, which views current interpersonal and emotional experience as having been influenced by early childhood experience (Bibring 1952). Revised conceptualizations have emphasized how relationships are internalized and transformed into a sense of self (e.g., Kohut and Wolf 1978; Mahler 1952). Psychopathology is theorized as being related to arrestments in the development of the self, and depression is viewed as a symptom state resulting from unresolved intrapsychic conflict that may be activated by life events such as loss. During therapy, patients are encouraged to develop insight into past experiences and how these experiences influence their current relationships.

CBT techniques currently in use generally combine earlier work that used either solely cognitive or solely behavioral therapies and now encompass a wide variety of treatment protocols. Cognitive therapies focus on problematic thoughts that may perpetuate depression. The goal is to change and adapt cognitive patterns away from negative thoughts that have become automatic. By changing the thoughts, therapists hope to change underlying dysfunctional attitudes that are hypothesized to result in relapse (Floyd and Scogin 1998). **(pp. 522, 524, 525)**

29.3 Investigators have studied the effects of exercise on depression in older adults. In one study, supervised exercise therapy, medication alone, and combined exercise and medication were evaluated to determine their effectiveness in treating depression in older adults. What was one of the results of this study?

   A. Medication alone was superior to supervised exercise therapy or combined exercise and medication therapy.
   B. Supervised exercise therapy was superior to medication alone or combined exercise and medication therapy.
   C. Combined exercise and medication therapy was superior to either medication alone or supervised exercise therapy.
   D. Follow-up assessments at 10 months revealed lower rates of depression in the medication group than in the supervised exercise therapy group or the combined treatment group.
   E. There were no significant differences among treatment groups.

The correct response is option E.

Using a form of behavioral activation, Blumenthal et al. (1999) studied the effects of exercise on depression in older adults. Supervised exercise therapy, medication (sertraline) alone, or combined exercise and medication therapy all produced significant improvements in depressive symptoms. There were no significant differences between treatment groups, which suggests that exercise training might be comparable with the use of medication in older adults. Interestingly, follow-up assessment at 10 months showed lower rates of depression in the exercise-training group than in the medication or combined treatment groups (Babyak et al. 2000). **(p. 522)**

29.4 Among older adults, the most commonly diagnosed anxiety disorder (believed to be underdiagnosed in older adults) is

   A. Panic disorder.
   B. Acute stress disorder.
   C. Social phobia.
   D. Generalized anxiety disorder (GAD).
   E. Obsessive-compulsive disorder.

The correct response is option D.

Among older adults, GAD is the most commonly diagnosed anxiety disorder. On the basis of data in Epidemiologic Catchment Area surveys, it is estimated that up to 1.9% of older adults currently experience GAD (Blazer et al. 1991). Although researchers tend to agree that rates of GAD are lower in older adults than in younger populations, several researchers have suggested that GAD is still underdiagnosed in this population (Palmer et al. 1997; Stanley and Novy 2000). Diagnostic criteria for GAD in younger adults may fail to take into account different ways that older adults experience anxiety. Older adults may focus on different targets of worry and on somatic symptoms that can be confused with medical illness (Sable and Jeste 2001). Evidence also suggests that GAD often appears in conjunction with depressive symptoms, which confuses both diagnostic criteria and the focal point for treatment strategies. One study reported that 91% of older adults with GAD diagnoses also met criteria for depression (Lindesay et al. 1989). The problems of variant symptom presentations, overemphasis on somatic symptoms, and depressive comorbidity create confusion in both diagnoses and treatment choices. (p. 528)

29.5   The rate of personality disorder among depressed older adult samples has been estimated to be

    A. 5%.
    B. 10%.
    C. 15%.
    D. 20%.
    E. 30%.

The correct response is option E.

Meta-analyses have concluded that the prevalence rate of personality disorder is between 10% and 20% of the older adult community (Abrams 1996; Abrams and Horowitz 1999), essentially analogous to the 13% prevalence rate among younger age groups (Torgersen et al. 2001). Overall, the emotionally constricted/risk-averse disorders in clusters A (i.e., paranoid personality disorder, schizoid personality disorder) and C (i.e., obsessive-compulsive personality disorder, avoidant personality disorder, dependent personality disorder) are the most commonly diagnosed in late life (Abrams 1996; Abrams and Horowitz 1999; Kenan et al. 2000; Morse and Lynch 2004), and there are also high rates of the Not Otherwise Specified category compared with other individual personality disorder diagnoses (Abrams 1996; Abrams and Horowitz 1999; Kenan et al. 2000). In addition, personality disorder rates are even higher (approximately 30%) among depressed older adult samples (Abrams 1996; Thompson et al. 1988). Older adult depressed patients with comorbid personality disorder are four times more likely to experience maintenance or reemergence of depressive symptoms compared with those without personality disorder diagnoses (Morse and Lynch 2004). Despite this, with the exception of case studies, only one published outcome study has specifically focused on treating late-life personality disorders (Lynch et al. 2007). (p. 530)

References

Abrams RC: Personality disorders in the elderly. Int J Geriatr Psychiatry 11:759–763, 1996

Abrams RC, Horowitz SV: Personality disorders after age 50: a meta-analytic review of the literature, in Personality Disorders in Older Adults: Emerging Issues in Diagnosis and Treatment. Edited by Rosowsky E, Abrams RC. Mahwah, NJ, Erlbaum, 1999, pp 55–68

Babyak M, Blumenthal JA, Herman S, et al: Exercise treatment for major depression: maintenance of therapeutic benefit at 10 months. Psychosom Med 62:633–638, 2000

Bibring E: [The problem of depression.] Psyche 6:81–101, 1952

Blazer D, George LK, Hughes D: The epidemiology of anxiety disorders: an age comparison, in Anxiety in the Elderly: Treatment and Research. Edited by Salzman C, Lebowitz BD. New York, Springer, 1991, pp 17–30

Blumenthal JAP, Babyak MAP, Moore KAP, et al: Effects of exercise training on older patients with major depression. Arch Intern Med 159:2349–2356, 1999

Floyd M, Scogin F: Cognitive-behavior therapy for older adults: how does it work? Psychotherapy 35:459–463, 1998

Hinrichsen GA: Interpersonal psychotherapy for depressed older adults. J Geriatr Psychiatry 30:239–257, 1997

Kenan MM, Kendjelic EM, Molinari VA, et al: Age-related differences in the frequency of personality disorders among inpatient veterans. Int J Geriatr Psychiatry 15:831–837, 2000

Kohut H, Wolf ES: The disorders of the self and their treatment: an outline. Int J Psychoanal 59:413–425, 1978

Lindesay J, Briggs K, Murphy E: The Guy's/Age Concern Survey: prevalence rates of cognitive impairment, depression and anxiety in an urban elderly community. Br J Psychiatry 155:317–329, 1989

Lynch TR, Cheavens JS, Cukrowicz KC, et al: Treatment of older adults with co-morbid personality disorder and depression: a dialectical behavior therapy approach. Int J Geriatr Psychiatry 22:131–143, 2007

Mahler MS: On child psychosis and schizophrenia: autistic and symbiotic infantile psychoses. Psychoanal Study Child 7:286–305, 1952

Morse JQ, Lynch TR: A preliminary investigation of self-reported personality disorders in late life: prevalence, predictors of depressive severity, and clinical correlates. Aging Ment Health 8:307–315, 2004

Nezu AM: A problem-solving formulation of depression: a literature review and proposal of a pluralistic model. Clin Psychol Rev 7:121–144, 1987

Palmer BW, Jeste DV, Sheikh JI: Anxiety disorders in the elderly: DSM-IV and other barriers to diagnosis and treatment. J Affect Disord 46:183–190, 1997

Reynolds CF 3rd, Frank E, Perel JM, et al: Nortriptyline and interpersonal psychotherapy as maintenance therapies for recurrent major depression: a randomized controlled trial in patients older than 59 years. JAMA 281:39–45, 1999

Sable JA, Jeste DV: Anxiety disorders in older adults. Curr Psychiatr Rep 3:302–307, 2001

Stanley MA, Novy DM: Cognitive-behavior therapy for generalized anxiety in late life: an evaluative overview. J Anxiety Disord 14:191–207, 2000

Thompson LW, Gallagher D: Efficacy of psychotherapy in the treatment of late-life depression. Advances in Behaviour Research and Therapy 6:127–139, 1984

Thompson LW, Coon DW, Gallagher-Thompson D, et al: Comparison of desipramine and cognitive/behavioral therapy in the treatment of elderly outpatients with mild-to-moderate depression. Am J Geriatr Psychiatry 9:225–240, 2001

Thompson LW, Gallagher D, Czirr R: Personality disorder and outcome in the treatment of late-life depression. J Geriatr Psychiatry 21:133–146, 1988

Torgersen S, Kringlen E, Cramer V: The prevalence of personality disorders in a community sample. Arch Gen Psychiatry 58: 590–596, 2001

Chapter 30

Working With Families of Older Adults

Select the single best response for each question.

30.1 For psychiatrists and other mental health professionals working with families, there are a number of clinical reminders that may prove useful. Which of the following is one of those clinical reminders?

    A. The family is frequently the obstacle to effective care for the older member.

    B. Different perceptions and expectations of close and distant family members do not necessarily result in family conflict.

    C. Denial on the part of family members must be confronted.

    D. A family caregiver's awareness of an available service invariably leads to appropriate use of that service.

    E. A primary caregiver at home is efficient and preferred.

The correct response is option E.

The following clinical reminders about family care may prove useful in working with families of older adults:

1. Family care is an adaptive challenge: the family is not necessarily the problem, nor is the family necessarily the obstacle to effective care.

2. The family rarely has one voice. Different perceptions and expectations of close and distant family members frequently precipitate family conflict.

3. Few families have the luxury of one person needing care at a time. There is much less manipulation by dependent elders than there are real unmet dependency needs.

4. There is no one right way or ideal place to offer family care. Many families are forced to choose between equally unacceptable options.

5. Successful family caregivers are flexible in adjusting expectations of themselves, the older adult, and other family members as they work to fit the needs and capacities of all.

6. Families caring for older adults with dementia must define and negotiate complex situations, perform physically intimate tasks, manage emotions and communication, modify expectations, and capitalize on the older adult's preserved capacities.

7. A family caregiver's awareness of an available service, need for the service, or knowledge of how to access the service does not necessarily lead to appropriate or timely use of that service.

8. There is no perfect control in a family care situation. Families are better off if they work on their reactions to stress or lack of control.

9. Denial is a common defense of family caregivers. Some people need to deny the inevitable outcome (loss of a beloved spouse or eventual placement of a parent in a nursing home) to provide hopeful, consistent daily care.

10. A primary caregiver at home is efficient and preferred. Primary caregivers need breaks, respite, backup people, and services to supplement their personalized care. Even in ideal situations, contingency plans are necessary. (pp. 540–541)

30.2 Clinical goals for psychiatrists and other mental health professionals working with families of older adults will vary depending on presenting problems and family resources. However, some common goals are applicable to most families. All of the following are examples of these common clinical goals *except*

    A. To address safety issues.
    B. To help family members care for their elder member without needing outside help.
    C. To mobilize secondary family support.
    D. To facilitate appropriate decision making at care transitions.
    E. To normalize variability.

The correct response is option B.

Clinical goals with families of older adults will vary with presenting problems and family resources. Common goals, however, are to normalize variability, address safety issues, mobilize secondary family support, facilitate appropriate decision making at care transitions, and help family members accept help or let go of direct care as necessary. In essence, the family is forced to adapt to a new state of "normal" in their family life, often with resistance from the member with dementia. Well-timed psychiatric help in interpreting the family's and the elder's reluctance to accept new realities can promote appropriate decision making and help smooth care transitions. **(p. 541)**

30.3 Families have certain expectations of psychiatrists. Which of the following is one of these expectations?

    A. Families want action from psychiatrists and not listening.
    B. Psychiatrists should not ask what else is going on in the family's lives since they already have much to deal with.
    C. Families appreciate general suggestions from psychiatrists to take care of themselves.
    D. Families look to psychiatrists for support in making certain decisions.
    E. Psychiatrists should discourage family members from expressing their feelings.

The correct response is option D.

Families look to psychiatrists for support in making certain decisions and may ask for help in mobilizing other family members.

Families want psychiatrists to listen without rushing to implied understanding or suggestions. Families of older adults expect to be asked what they have tried in coping with their relative's impairment. Even more, these families appreciate the psychiatrist's asking about what else is going on in their lives.

Families of older adults want psychiatrists to tailor information and education relevant to their immediate, pressing concerns.

When depleted primary caregivers are confronting the range of behavioral symptoms of older adults with Alzheimer's disease, they may look to the psychiatrist to lend energy, a proactive attitude and perspective, and objectivity. They want acknowledgment of their contributions to the older adult's quality of life or absolution and forgiveness for what they were unable to achieve despite their best intentions.

Families also appreciate preventive self-care reminders from psychiatrists, but vague suggestions that caregivers need to take care of themselves often frustrate overwhelmed families that have few resources (Burton et al. 1997). Family members need help translating principles of respite in ways that are congruent with their personal values and cultural expectations.

Family caregivers expect psychiatrists to let them express feelings, even when these feelings are judged to be unacceptable. **(pp. 543–544)**

30.4 It is important for the psychiatrist to assess the family of an older adult. All of the following are examples of effective assessment *except*

  A. Asking about other family commitments.
  B. Carefully assessing cultural expectations.
  C. Avoiding asking about previous and current help from family members.
  D. Assessing family strengths, skills, and goals.
  E. Asking the family to describe a typical day.

The correct response is option C.

Assessment should include some review of the family's experience with previous and current help from family members or paid services. Some key questions include the adequacy, quality, cost, and dependability of the help.

One of the most useful ways to elicit a picture of family functioning is to ask the family to describe a typical day. It is wise to assess the home and neighborhood environment. The psychiatrist should ask specifically about the primary caregiver's health. Another key to effective family assessment is to ask about other family commitments. Cultural expectations must be carefully assessed along with each family member's subjective perceptions of financial resources. It is wise to assess family strengths, skills, and goals. **(pp. 544–545)**

30.5 There are a number of key messages that psychiatrists should convey to family caregivers over time. Which of the following is one of these messages?

  A. You can only do what is best at the time. Doubts will occur.
  B. Avoid expressing your honest feelings to anyone since your conversation may get back to the older adult.
  C. Try not to compromise among competing needs, loyalties, or commitments. Make firm commitments.
  D. Save your time and energy to celebrate major, not minor, successes.
  E. The older adult may often be unhappy with what you have done.

The correct response is option A.

Some key messages to convey to family caregivers include:

  1. Be willing to listen to the older adult, but understand that you cannot fix or do everything he or she may want or need.
  2. You are living with a situation you did not create, and your choices are limited by circumstances beyond your control.
  3. You can only do what seems best at the time. Identify what you can and will tolerate, then set limits and call in reinforcements. Doubts are inevitable.
  4. Find someone with whom you can be brutally honest, express those feelings, and move on.
  5. Solving problems is much easier than living with the solutions. It is tempting for distant relatives to second guess or criticize. Hope for the best but plan for the worst.
  6. It is not always possible to compare how one person handles things with how another relative would handle them if the positions were reversed.
  7. The older adult is not unhappy or upset because of what you have done. He or she is living with unwanted dependency.
  8. Considering what is best for your family involves compromise among competing needs, loyalties, and commitments.
  9. Find ways to let your older relative give to or help you. He or she needs to feel purposeful, appreciated, and loved.
  10. Take time to celebrate small victories when things go well. **(p. 547)**

Reference

Burton LC, Newsom JT, Schultz R, et al: Preventive health behaviors among spousal caregivers. Prev Med 26:162–169, 1997

Chapter 31

Clinical Psychiatry in the Nursing Home

Select the single best response for each question.

31.1 Epidemiological studies during the 1980s and 1990s reported prevalence rates for psychiatric disorders among nursing home residents. On the basis of psychiatric interviews of nursing home patients in randomly selected samples, investigators reported rates for psychiatric disorders in which of the following ranges?

    A. 50%–55%.
    B. 60%–65%.
    C. 70%–75%.
    D. 80%–85%.
    E. 90%–95%.

The correct response is option E.

Epidemiological studies conducted between 1986 and 1993 uniformly reported high prevalence rates for psychiatric disorders among nursing home residents. Rovner et al. (1990) reported the prevalence of psychiatric disorders among persons newly admitted to a proprietary chain of nursing homes to be 80.2%. Parmelee et al. (1989) found psychiatric disorders diagnosed according to DSM-III-R (American Psychiatric Association 1987) criteria in 91% of the residents of a large urban geriatric center. On the basis of psychiatric interviews of subjects in randomly selected samples, other investigators found prevalence rates of DSM-III (American Psychiatric Association 1980) or DSM-III-R disorders to be as high as 94% (Chandler and Chandler 1988; Rovner et al. 1986; Tariot et al. 1993). Although some studies reported lower rates, those investigations used less rigorous methods for sampling or diagnosis (Burns et al. 1988; Custer et al. 1984; German et al. 1986; National Center for Health Statistics 1987; Teeter et al. 1976). In one study, case ascertainment by review of selected medical records revealed a 68% prevalence of psychiatric diagnosis (Linkins et al. 2006), suggesting that chart documentation of mental disorders by nursing home clinicians may underestimate the actual rates of mental disorders. **(p. 554)**

31.2 Dementia is the most common psychiatric disorder in nursing home patients. What is the second most common psychiatric disorder?

    A. Generalized anxiety disorder.
    B. Depression.
    C. Schizophrenia.
    D. Bipolar disorder.
    E. Alcoholism.

The correct response is option B.

Among community-dwelling elders in the United States and Europe, depression increases the risk of nursing home admission (Ahmed et al. 2007; Harris and Cooper 2006; Onder et al. 2007), and this association remains after controlling for age, physical illness, and functional status (Harris 2007). Among those who reside in nursing homes, depressive disorders represent the second most common psychiatric diagnosis. Most studies in U.S. nursing homes show depression prevalence rates of 15%–50%, depending on the population studied and the instruments used, whether major depression or depressive symptoms are being reported, and whether primary depression and depression occurring secondary to dementia are considered together or separately (Baker and Miller 1991; Chandler and Chandler 1988; Hyer and Blazer 1982; Katz et al. 1989; Kaup et al. 2007; Lesher 1986; Levin et al. 2007; Parmelee et al. 1989; Rovner et al. 1986, 1990, 1991; Tariot et al. 1993; Teeter et al. 1976). Studies from other countries have shown similar rates (Ames 1990, 1991; Ames et al. 1988; Chahine et al. 2007; Harrison et al. 1990; Horiguchi and Inami 1991; Jongenelis et al. 2004; Mann et al. 1984; Snowdon 1986; Snowdon and Donnelly 1986; Spagnoli et al. 1986; Trichard et al. 1982). Thus, the high rates of depression in the United States cannot be attributed solely to problems in this country's approach to long-term care for elderly persons. (pp. 555–556)

31.3 A number of nonpharmacological interventions have proven to be effective in reducing agitation in nursing home patients. Which of the following has *not* been shown to be effective in reducing agitation?

 A. Daytime physical activity combined with a nighttime program to decrease noise and sleep-disruptive nursing care practices.
 B. Activities matched to skills and interest of patients.
 C. Bright light therapy.
 D. Individualized modification in the physical environment.
 E. Individualized consultation for staff nurses about the management of patients with dementia.

The correct response is option C.

Bright light therapy has been shown to increase observed nocturnal sleep time, but not to improve agitated behavior in nursing home residents with dementia (Lyketsos et al. 1999).

Reductions in agitation were observed in a study of a daytime physical activity intervention combined with a nighttime program to decrease noise and sleep-disruptive nursing care practices (Alessi 1999).

Activities matched to skills and interests of residents with dementia have been shown to reduce agitation and negative affect (Kolanowski et al. 2005).

Other programs decrease behavioral difficulties through individualized modifications in the physical environment (van Weert et al. 2005).

Individualized consultation for staff nurses about the management of patients with dementia was also shown to diminish the use of physical restraints (Evans et al. 1997). (p. 557)

31.4 Efficacy of some of the atypical antipsychotic agents for the treatment of psychotic symptoms and agitated behavior in nursing home residents without dementia has been demonstrated in several multicenter randomized, double-blind, placebo-controlled clinical trials. Which of the following agents has *not* been studied in this manner?

 A. Aripiprazole.
 B. Olanzapine.
 C. Quetiapine.
 D. Risperidone.
 E. Ziprasidone.

The correct response is option E.

Some of the earlier studies provided evidence for the efficacy of antipsychotic drugs in managing agitation and related symptoms in nursing home residents with dementia, but the effect sizes were often modest, and high placebo response rates were common (Barnes et al. 1982; Schneider et al. 1990; Sunderland and Silver 1988). Subsequently, several multicenter, randomized, double-blind, placebo-controlled clinical trials demonstrated efficacy of some of the atypical antipsychotic agents for the treatment of psychotic symptoms and agitated behavior in nursing home residents with dementia. These include published studies of risperidone (Brodaty et al. 2003; Katz et al. 1999), olanzapine (Meehan et al. 2002; Street et al. 2000), quetiapine (Zhong et al. 2007), and aripiprazole (Mintzer et al. 2007). (p. 561)

31.5 Analyses of safety data from randomized, controlled studies of atypical antipsychotic drugs in elderly patients with dementia revealed significantly increased risks of cerebrovascular adverse events and mortality. Which of the following agents had the highest rate of cerebrovascular adverse events?

    A. Aripiprazole.
    B. Olanzapine.
    C. Quetiapine.
    D. Risperidone.
    E. Ziprasidone.

The correct response is option D.

Since 2003, analyses of safety data from randomized, controlled studies of atypical antipsychotic drugs in elderly patients with dementia have revealed significantly increased risks of cerebrovascular adverse events and mortality in this population. Although elevated risks were not found in every study, pooled analyses showed that the rate of cerebrovascular adverse events (including stroke and transient ischemic attacks) is greater than placebo by 2.3% in elderly patients treated with risperidone, 0.9% in patients treated with olanzapine, and 0.7% in those treated with aripiprazole. Most of the affected individuals had known cerebrovascular risk factors prior to starting drug treatment. These findings led to regulatory warnings in the United States, Canada, and the United Kingdom regarding the safety of these drugs in elderly patients with dementia. (p. 568)

31.6 Although selective serotonin reuptake inhibitors (SSRIs) generally are well tolerated by frail elderly nursing home patients, this class of antidepressants has been associated with which of the following adverse events?

    A. Falls.
    B. Strokes.
    C. Diabetes.
    D. Delirium.
    E. Hypertension.

The correct response is option A.

Although the SSRIs might be expected to be well tolerated by frail elderly nursing home patients because of their side-effect profile, there is evidence that these drugs can cause serious adverse events in this population. Thapa et al. (1998) demonstrated that the use of SSRIs was associated with a nearly twofold increase in the risk of falls in nursing home residents, comparable to the risk found with tricyclic antidepressant drugs. Investigators in the United Kingdom reported that antidepressant use was associated with better physical functioning but also with greater frequency of falls in residential care patients (Arthur et al. 2002). (p. 569)

31.7 Regulations promulgated by the Health Care Financing Administration require that nursing home residents not receive unnecessary drugs. An unnecessary drug is defined by all of the following *except*

   A. Excessive duration.
   B. Inadequate dose.
   C. Without adequate monitoring.
   D. Without adequate indications.
   E. In the presence of adverse consequences.

The correct response is option B.

An unnecessary drug is defined as any drug used 1) in excessive dose (including duplicate therapy), 2) for excessive duration, 3) without adequate monitoring, 4) without adequate indications for its use, 5) in the presence of adverse consequences that indicate that it should be reduced or discontinued, or 6) for any combination of the first five reasons (Health Care Financing Administration 1991). **(p. 569)**

References

Ahmed A, Lefante CM, Alam N: Depression and nursing home admission among hospitalized older adults with coronary artery disease: a propensity score analysis. Am J Geriatr Cardiol 16:76–83, 2007

Alessi CA: A randomized trial of a combined physical activity and environmental intervention in nursing home residents: do sleep and agitation improve? J Am Geriatr Soc 47:784–791, 1999

American Psychiatric Association: Diagnostic and Statistical Manual of Mental Disorders, 3rd Edition. Washington, DC, American Psychiatric Association, 1980

American Psychiatric Association: Diagnostic and Statistical Manual of Mental Disorders, 3rd Edition Revised. Washington, DC, American Psychiatric Association, 1987

Ames D: Depression among elderly residents of local-authority residential homes: its nature and the efficacy of intervention. Br J Psychiatry 156:667–675, 1990

Ames D: Epidemiological studies of depression among the elderly in residential and nursing homes. Int J Geriatr Psychiatry 6:347–354, 1991

Ames D, Ashby D, Mann AH, et al: Psychiatric illness in elderly residents of part III homes in one London borough: prognosis and review. Age Ageing 17:249–256, 1988

Arthur A, Matthews R, Jagger C, et al: Factors associated with antidepressant treatment in residential care: changes between 1990 and 1997. Int J Geriatr Psychiatry 17:54–60, 2002

Baker FM, Miller CL: Screening a skilled nursing home population for depression. J Geriatr Psychiatry Neurol 4:218–221, 1991

Barnes R, Veith R, Okimoto J, et al: Efficacy of antipsychotic medications in behaviorally disturbed dementia patients. Am J Psychiatry 139:1170–1174, 1982

Brodaty H, Ames D, Snowdon J, et al: A randomized placebo-controlled trial of risperidone for the treatment of aggression, agitation, and psychosis of dementia. J Clin Psychiatry 64:134–143, 2003

Burns BJ, Larson DB, Goldstrom ID, et al: Mental disorder among nursing home patients: preliminary findings from the National Nursing Home Survey Pretest. Int J Geriatr Psychiatry 3:27–35, 1988

Chahine LM, Bijlsma A, Hospers AP, et al: Dementia and depression among nursing home residents in Lebanon: a pilot study. Int J Geriatr Psychiatry 22:283–285, 2007

Chandler JD, Chandler JE: The prevalence of neuropsychiatric disorders in a nursing home population. J Geriatr Psychiatry Neurol 1:71–76, 1988

Custer RL, Davis JE, Gee SC: Psychiatric drug usage in VA nursing home care units. Psychiatr Ann 14:285–292, 1984

Evans LK, Strumpf NE, Allen-Taylor SL, et al: A clinical trial to reduce restraints in nursing homes. J Am Geriatr Soc 45:675–681, 1997

German PS, Shapiro S, Kramer M: Nursing home study of eastern Baltimore epidemiologic catchment area, in Mental Illness in Nursing Homes: Agenda for Research. Edited by Harper MS, Lebowitz BD. Rockville, MD, National Institute of Mental Health, 1986, pp 21–40

Harris Y: Depression as a risk factor for nursing home admission among older individuals. J Am Med Dir Assoc 8:14–20, 2007

Harris Y, Cooper JK: Depressive symptoms in older people predict nursing home admission. J Am Geriatr Soc 54:593–597, 2006

Health Care Financing Administration: Medicare and Medicaid: Requirements for Long Term Care Facilities, Final Regulations. Fed Regist 56:48865–48921, 1991

Horiguchi J, Inami Y: A survey of the living conditions and psychological states of elderly people admitted to nursing homes in Japan. Acta Psychiatr Scand 83:338–341, 1991

Hyer L, Blazer DG: Depressive symptoms: impact and problems in long term care facilities. International Journal of Behavioral Gerontology 1:33–44, 1982

Jongenelis K, Pot AM, Eisses AM, et al: Prevalence and risk indicators of depression in elderly nursing home patients: the AGED study. J Affect Disord 83:135–142, 2004

Katz IR, Lesher E, Kleban M, et al: Clinical features of depression in the nursing home. Int Psychogeriatr 1:5–15, 1989

Katz IR, Jeste DV, Mintzer JE, et al: Comparison of risperidone and placebo for psychosis and behavioral disturbances associated with dementia: a randomized, double-blind trial. J Clin Psychiatry 60:107–115, 1999

Kaup BA, Loreck D, Gruber-Baldini AL, et al: Depression and its relationship to function and medical status, by dementia status, in nursing home admissions. Am J Geriatr Psychiatry 15:438–442, 2007

Kolanowski AM, Litaker M, Buettner L: Efficacy of theory-based activities for behavioral symptoms of dementia. Nurs Res 54:219–228, 2005

Lesher E: Validation of the Geriatric Depression Scale among nursing home residents. Clinics in Gerontology 4:21–28, 1986

Levin CA, Wei W, Akincigil A, et al: Prevalence and treatment of diagnosed depression among elderly nursing home residents in Ohio. J Am Med Dir Assoc 8:585–594, 2007

Linkins KW, Lucca AM, Housman M, et al: Use of PASRR programs to assess serious mental illness and service access in nursing homes. Psychiatr Serv 57:325–332, 2006

Lyketsos CG, Lindell Veiel L, Baker A, et al: A randomized, controlled trial of bright light therapy for agitated behaviors in dementia patients residing in long-term care. Int J Geriatr Psychiatry 14:520–525, 1999

Mann AH, Graham N, Ashby D: Psychiatric illness in residential homes for the elderly: a survey in one London borough. Age Ageing 13:257–265, 1984

Meehan KM, Wang H, David SR, et al: Comparison of rapidly acting intramuscular olanzapine, lorazepam, and placebo: a double-blind, randomized study in acutely agitated patients with dementia. Neuropsychopharmacology 26:494–504, 2002

Mintzer JE, Tune LE, Breder CD, et al: Aripiprazole for the treatment of psychoses in institutionalized patients with Alzheimer dementia: a multicenter, randomized, double-blind, placebo-controlled assessment of three fixed doses. Am J Geriatr Psychiatry 15:918–931, 2007

National Center for Health Statistics: Use of Nursing Homes by the Elderly: Preliminary Data From the 1985 National Nursing Home Survey (DHHS Publ No PHS-87-1250). Hyattsville, MD, National Center for Health Statistics, 1987

Onder G, Liperoti R, Soldato M, et al: Depression and risk of nursing home admission among older adults in home care in Europe: results from the Aged in Home Care (AdHOC) study. J Clin Psychiatry 68:1392–1398, 2007

Parmelee PA, Katz IR, Lawton MP: Depression among institutionalized aged: assessment and prevalence estimation. J Gerontol 44:M22–M29, 1989

Rovner BW, Kafonek S, Filipp L, et al: Prevalence of mental illness in a community nursing home. Am J Psychiatry 143:1446–1449, 1986

Rovner BW, German PS, Broadhead J, et al: The prevalence and management of dementia and other psychiatric disorders in nursing homes. Int Psychogeriatr 2:13–24, 1990

Rovner BW, German PS, Brant LJ, et al: Depression and mortality in nursing homes. JAMA 265:993–996, 1991

Schneider LS, Pollock VE, Lyness SA: A meta-analysis of controlled trials of neuroleptic treatment in dementia. J Am Geriatr Soc 38:553–563, 1990

Snowdon J: Dementia, depression, and life satisfaction in nursing homes. Int J Geriatr Psychiatry 1:85–91, 1986

Snowdon J, Donnelly N: A study of depression in nursing homes. J Psychiatr Res 20:327–333, 1986

Spagnoli A, Foresti G, Macdonald A, et al: Dementia and depression in Italian geriatric institutions. Int J Geriatr Psychiatry 1:15–23, 1986

Street JS, Clark WS, Gannon KS, et al: Olanzapine treatment of psychotic and behavioral symptoms in patients with Alzheimer disease in nursing care facilities: a double-blind, randomized, placebo-controlled trial. Arch Gen Psychiatry 57:968–976, 2000

Sunderland T, Silver MA: Neuroleptics in the treatment of dementia. Int J Geriatr Psychiatry 3:79–88, 1988

Tariot PN, Podgorski CA, Blazina L, et al: Mental disorders in the nursing home: another perspective. Am J Psychiatry 150:1063–1069, 1993

Teeter RB, Garetz FK, Miller WR, et al: Psychiatric disturbances of aged patients in skilled nursing homes. Am J Psychiatry 133:1430–1434, 1976

Thapa PB, Gideon P, Cost CW, et al: Antidepressants and the risk of falls among nursing home residents. N Engl J Med 339:875–882, 1998

Trichard L, Zabow A, Gillis LS: Elderly persons in old age homes: a medical, psychiatric and social investigation. S Afr Med J 61:624–627, 1982

van Weert JC, van Dulmen AM, Spreeuwenberg PM, et al: Behavioral and mood effects of snoezelen integrated into 24-hour dementia care. J Am Geriatr Soc 53:24–33, 2005

Zhong KX, Tariot PN, Mintzer J, et al: Quetiapine to treat agitation in dementia: a randomized, double-blind, placebo-controlled study. Curr Alzheimer Res 4:81–93, 2007

Chapter 32

The Continuum of Caring in the Long Term

Movement Toward the Community

Select the single best response for each question.

32.1 In the U.S. population, disability that results in institutional care has been

A. Increasing at the rate of about 1% a year.
B. Increasing at the rate of about 5% a year.
C. Remaining constant.
D. Decreasing at the rate of about 1% a year.
E. Decreasing at the rate of about 5% a year.

The correct response is option D.

Confirming evidence indicates that disability in the U.S. population resulting in institutional care has apparently been declining at the rate of about 1% a year over the past several decades (Cutler 2001). And in the past decade the occupancy rate of available nursing home beds has continued to decline as alternative forms of supportive care in the community have increased (Smith 2003). **(p. 569)**

32.2 The most notable example of federal policy innovation in long-term care is the modification of Medicaid under the Reagan administration's home- and community-based care (HCBS) waivers. This provision

A. Excluded nursing homes from receiving Medicaid except under special circumstances.
B. Reduced funding for nursing homes.
C. Enabled states to seek waivers for home- and community-based options for older and disabled beneficiaries who normally would require nursing care.
D. Enabled states to seek waivers creating acute inpatient units for short stays for the older and disabled.
E. Excluded federal reimbursement for patients with psychiatric disorders who were admitted to nursing homes.

The correct response is option C.

Federal policy on long-term care has been slow to change. Beginning with federal devolution of responsibility for long-term care to states in the mid-1980s, federal interest focused on cost containment. Perhaps the most notable example of federal policy innovation in long-term care is the modification of Medicaid under the Reagan administration's HCBS waivers. This provision enabled states to seek waivers creating home- and community-based options for older and disabled beneficiaries who otherwise would require nursing home care. Federal approval of such waivers required states to document that Medicaid expenditures would be less than the expenses incurred if care were provided in nursing homes. With the impetus of HCBS waivers and growing state expenditures, the 1990s were years of growth in innovation of state long-term care policy as many states chose not to wait for further federal innovation. **(p. 589)**

32.3 Hospice care is designed to achieve a number of goals. Which of the following is **not** one of these goals?

    A. Maximize a sense of self-efficacy in individuals.
    B. Manage a terminal patient's final transition in a minimally medical environment.
    C. Provide social and emotional support to the patient.
    D. Create a sense of collective self-efficacy for families.
    E. Provide access to the latest technological innovations.

The correct response is option E.

Hospice care is designed to maximize a sense of self-efficacy in individuals and a sense of collective efficacy for families in managing as much as possible a terminal patient's final transition in a minimally medical environment and with the promise of a collective assurance that social and emotional support reliably will remain available. The life-prolonging high-technology interventions characteristic of hospitals are simply not available (by design), and this, economists have conjectured, is one likely explanation of why the cost of hospice remains relatively low when compared with hospitalization. **(p. 590)**

32.4 Consumer-directed care has been slower to develop among older adults primarily because of

    A. Lack of financial support for innovative alternatives.
    B. Concerns about whether older persons are capable.
    C. Concerns over increased possible costs of alternative services.
    D. Questions about the role of federal and state agencies.
    E. Lack of consensus as to what needs to be done.

The correct response is option B.

Programs of consumer-directed care vary widely across countries and across states in the United States. An overview article that displays with clarity the observed variety and issues is offered online by the Urban Institute (Tilly et al. 2000). Prominent issues when older consumers are involved include the competence of consumers to make decisions and manage finances, whether family members can be employed, whether cash and cash payments are under consumer controls, availability of consumer training for care direction, availability of appropriate care providers to be hired, and provision of quality assurance. Consumer-directed care has been slower to develop among older adults because of concerns about whether older persons are capable of directing their services and about how to assure the quality of care without agency oversight and accountability. Although definitive answers are not yet available for such issues, consumer-directed personal assistance services continue to flourish internationally and have achieved the endorsement of the National Council on Disability in the United States. **(pp. 591–592)**

32.5 The basic concepts of the distinctive philosophy of assisted-living housing include all of the following **except**

    A. Allowing families to have more decision-making authority.
    B. Matching services with individual need.
    C. Offering a private, self-contained space of one's own.
    D. Sharing responsibility for care among residents, family, and staff.
    E. Enhancing the availability to residents of information for informed choice.

The correct response is option A.

The four basic concepts of the distinctive philosophy of assisted-living housing in its ideal form are 1) offering a private, self-contained space of one's own, 2) matching reliably available services with measured individual need, 3) sharing responsibility for care among residents, family, and staff, and 4) enhancing in residents the availability of information for informed choice and control of their lives. **(p. 592)**

32.6 In health services research on mental health in the United States, the major issue that is discussed often and early is

    A. Access concerns.
    B. The role of primary care physicians.
    C. Making an accurate diagnosis.
    D. Costs.
    E. Evidence-based practices.

The correct response is option D.

In health services research on mental health in the United States, the issue of cost tends to be raised early and often. Discussion of mental health care in one of the most prestigious journals has focused on economic issues such as 1) concern of employers underwriting health care for employees that demand for mental health services might be limitless, 2) concern of consumers and consumer advocates that insurance for mental health care might be arbitrarily limited, and 3) concern of ethicists that mental health services, already marginalized and undercapitalized in the dominant medicalized care system, may, in the interest of cost control, be even more inequitably treated. One symptom of the current interest in cost control of mental health services is the practice of "carving out" of such services from managed care insurance. This practice refers to contracting with "behavioral health" companies specifically to manage mental health services. This practice has demonstrably reduced costs by limiting the number of services provided and by limiting days in the hospital. **(p. 593)**

References

Cutler DM: Declining disability among the elderly. Health Aff 20:1–27, 2001
Smith D: Reinventing Care: Assisted Living in New York City. Nashville, TN, Vanderbilt University Press, 2003
Tilly J, Wiener J, Cueller A: Consumer-directed home and community care in five countries: policy issues for older adults and government. October 2000. Available at http://www.urban.org/publications/410330.html. Accessed March 3, 2008.

C h a p t e r 3 3

Legal, Ethical, and Policy Issues

Select the single best response for each question.

33.1 The Omnibus Budget Reconciliation Act of 1987 (OBRA-87) made a number of changes to how Medicare covered outpatient psychiatric services. Which of the following changes occurred as a result of this legislation?

  A. Allowed licensed clinical psychologists to bill Medicare for mental health services.
  B. Changed the copayment for psychotherapy services from 50% to 20%.
  C. Raised the cap for psychiatry reimbursement to $2,200.
  D. Eliminated the cap on outpatient mental health services.
  E. Allowed licensed certified social workers to bill Medicare for mental health services.

The correct response is option C.

Between 1966 and 1988, Medicare Part B covered outpatient psychiatric services up to a maximum of $500, subject to a 50% copayment; thus, Medicare paid only $250 per year. OBRA-87 raised the $500 cap for psychotherapy reimbursement to $2,200 per year but retained the 50% copayment, thereby limiting actual Medicare payments to $1,100 per year. However, medical management of psychotropic medications was exempted from this limit, and the copayment for these services was reduced to 20% under OBRA-87. Although the Omnibus Budget Reconciliation Act of 1989 eliminated the cap on outpatient mental health services, the 50% copayment was retained for psychotherapy services, and that disparity with coverage for general medical care (which requires only a 20% copayment) remains as a matter of dispute in Congress today. Consumer and professional groups have lobbied to change this discriminatory policy.

In 1990, the Medicare Part B psychiatric benefit was expanded to allow licensed clinical psychologists and certified social workers to bill Medicare for mental health services. **(p. 604)**

33.2 Between the years of 1990 and 2000, a number of changes occurred in the demographic characteristics of veterans receiving mental health services from the Department of Veterans Affairs (VA). Which of the following was one of these changes?

  A. There was a fourfold decrease in the number of veterans ages 75–84 who received mental health services.
  B. The most rapid increase in demand for services was from younger veterans (ages 35–44).
  C. Fewer than 5 million veterans are over age 65.
  D. The number of veterans ages 45–54 years who received mental health services more than tripled.
  E. The number of Vietnam-era veterans receiving mental health services is declining each year.

The correct response is option D.

A major provider of geriatric mental health care for older Americans is the VA health care system. More than 9 million veterans are older than age 65, and 510,000 are age 85 or older. The VA supports an extensive system of care for older adults with mental disorders, including acute inpatient psychiatric hospitalization, outpatient mental health and substance abuse clinics, a network of more than 120 long-term care facilities, and domiciliary care. Between 1990 and 2000, the number of veterans ages 45–54 who received mental health services from the

VA more than tripled. These were mostly Vietnam-era veterans, many of them the baby boomers who are now beginning to, and will continue to, swell the ranks of those who require geriatric care. However, the most rapid growth in demand during the same period was among the oldest of older veterans. From 1990 to 2000, the number of veterans ages 75–84 who received VA mental health services increased fourfold. **(p. 606)**

33.3 Numerous reviews and professional organizations' position statements have set forth guidelines for what constitutes good care at the end of life. Some common fundamentals have emerged. All of the following are examples of these fundamentals *except*

   A. Education and training of both professional and informal caregivers.
   B. Support of family and caregivers before and after the death of the patient.
   C. Maximizing quality of life.
   D. Removal of regulatory barriers to access care.
   E. Delay of advance planning and preparation for death, with a focus instead on the here and now.

The correct response is option E.

Numerous reviews and professional organizations' position statements have set forth guidelines for what constitutes good care at the end of life (American Geriatrics Society Ethics Committee 2007; Institute of Medicine 1997; Rabow et al. 2000; Sachs 2000). Despite considerable progress in recognizing the importance of quality of care for the dying, there is uncertainty and poor agreement about the characteristics of "the good death"; wide variation exists in attitudes among patients, physicians, other professional care providers, and family members concerning the specific attributes of this concept (Steinhauser et al. 2000). Nevertheless, some common fundamentals have emerged. Fundamental aspects for consideration when providing end-of-life care include 1) advance planning and preparation for death; 2) attention to quality of life, maximizing as many features as possible (including respect and dignity, autonomy, continuity of care, nonabandonment, alleviation of suffering of physical and mental symptoms, pain management, and spirituality); 3) support of family and caregivers before and after death of patient; 4) removal of regulatory barriers to facilitate access to care; and 5) education and training of both professional and informal caregivers. **(p. 609)**

33.4 A variety of techniques are available to psychiatrists to improve the quality of communication among patients, families, and health care professionals. Which of the following is *not* one of these techniques?

   A. Avoid clarifying vague terms so as not to make the patient more anxious.
   B. Identify a proxy decision maker.
   C. Identify patient concerns about the future.
   D. Learn the patient's understanding about potential outcomes.
   E. Learn about the patient's concept of quality of life.

The correct response is option A.

A variety of techniques are available to psychiatrists to improve the quality of communication between patients, families, and health care professionals. These techniques draw from the skills used for psychotherapy, with particular attention to permitting people to tell their stories. Such stories are the foundation for achieving common understandings of key issues such as the patient's prognosis, quality of life, and the goals of care. Useful questions to efficiently and effectively structure the "end-of-life" discussion with a patient (Karlawish et al. 1999) (Table 33–1) include 1) identifying the patient's present concerns, with attention to both the patient and the family; 2) learning the patient's understanding about potential outcomes; 3) correcting any misunderstandings of pertinent facts; 4) identifying the patient's concerns about the future; 5) identifying how the patient conceives of quality of life; 6) clarifying vague terms; and 7) identifying a proxy decision maker. **(pp. 610–611)**

TABLE 33–1. Questions to structure the end-of-life discussion with the patient

Identify the patient's present concerns, with attention to both the patient and the family.
    What concerns you most about your illness?
    How is treatment going for you? What about for your family?
    What has been most difficult about this illness for you? What about for your family?
Learn the patient's understanding about potential outcomes. Correct any misunderstandings of pertinent facts.
    When you think about your illness, what's the best that could happen?
    When you think about your illness, what's the worst that could happen?
Identify the patient's concerns about the future.
    What are your fears for the future?
    As you think about the future, what matters most to you?
Identify how the patient conceives of quality of life.
    If you were dying, where would you want to receive medical care? At home? In a hospital? In a hospice?
    What makes life worth living?
Clarify vague terms.
    What do you mean by "being a vegetable"?
Identify a proxy decision maker.
    If you were to become ill and could not speak for yourself like you are talking with me now, who would you want to speak
       on your behalf? Who do you trust?

Source. Adapted from Karlawish et al. 1999.

33.5 What is it called when a person makes a decision for a patient on the basis of what the patient's wishes would be were the patient capable of making the decision?

    A. Living will.
    B. Substituted judgment.
    C. Power of attorney.
    D. Guardianship.
    E. Durable power of attorney.

The correct response is option B.

When patients are unable to explicitly state their preferences, the process of *substituted judgment* should become operative. This means that another person makes a decision for a patient on the basis of what the patient's wishes would be if the patient were capable of making the decision. Several studies that have assessed the accuracy of substituted judgment have found what could be considered a disturbing result: poor congruence between patients' preferences and their spouses' and physicians' predictions of those preferences (see, e.g., Miles et al. 1996; Uhlmann 1988). However, these data are not on the whole as disturbing as they may seem. Sehgal et al. (1992) found that many patients, although capable of stating their advance directive for treatment, are willing to allow their trusted proxy to overrule this directive and do the opposite.

Advance directives for health care should include a *living will* and a *power of attorney for health care.* Power of attorney differs from guardianship in that the power of attorney is given by a competent individual, whereas the guardianship is imposed on a person who is deemed incompetent. A durable power of attorney takes effect when the person is unable to make the decisions the document addresses.

In many states, the living will relates only to 1) a terminal condition (incurable and irreversible) and 2) a permanently unconscious condition (persistent vegetative state). Hence, the living will is generally made in association with a durable power of attorney for health care, which confers wider scope for the decision-making right. (pp. 611–612)

References

American Geriatrics Society Ethics Committee: The Care of Dying Patients. New York, American Geriatrics Society, 2007. Available at: http://www.americangeriatrics.org/products/positionpapers/careofd.shtml. Accessed April 12, 2008

Institute of Medicine, Committee on Care at the End of Life: Approaching Death: Improving Care at the End of Life. Edited by Field MJ, Cassel CK. Washington, DC, National Academy Press, 1997

Karlawish JH, Quill T, Meier DE: A consensus-based approach to providing palliative care to patients who lack decision-making capacity. Ann Intern Med 130:835–840, 1999

Miles SH, Koepp R, Weber EP: Advance end-of-life treatment planning: a research review. Arch Intern Med 156:1062–1068, 1996

Omnibus Budget Reconciliation Act of 1987, Pub L No 100-203

Omnibus Budget Reconciliation Act of 1989, Pub L No 101-239

Rabow MW, Hardie GE, Fair JM, et al: End-of-life care content in 50 textbooks from multiple specialties. JAMA 283:771–778, 2000

Sachs GA: A piece of my mind: sometimes dying still stings. JAMA 284:2423, 2000

Sehgal A, Galbraith A, Chesney M, et al: How strictly do dialysis patients want their advance directive followed? JAMA 267:59–63, 1992

Steinhauser KE, Christakis NA, Clipp EC, et al: Factors considered important at the end of life by patients, family, physicians and other care providers. JAMA 284:2476–2482, 2000

Uhlmann RF, Pearlman RA, Cain KC: Physicians' and spouses' predictions of elderly patients' resuscitation preferences. J Gerontol 43:M115–M121, 1988

Chapter 34

The Past and Future of Geriatric Psychiatry

Select the single best response for each question.

34.1 Geriatric psychiatry faces special problems in obtaining referrals. Which is an example of one of these problems?

A. Inadequate training of geriatric psychiatrists to handle the referral questions.
B. Lack of need for specialized geriatric services.
C. Discouragement of referrals by managed care systems.
D. Improved training of primary care physicians to manage most problems.
E. Lack of demonstrated cost-effectiveness.

The correct response is option C.

Geriatric psychiatry faces special problems in the future regarding referrals. Managed care systems discourage referrals (although managed care penetration of Medicare is still limited), and geriatric psychiatry must help identify for the primary care physician the cases in which the unique skills of the geriatric psychiatrist can contribute to cost-effective care of the older adult. Although geriatric psychiatry is a broad-based specialty, in practice it rarely receives primary referrals. Patients do not usually consider the psychiatrist as the coordinator or the provider of general medical care. The geriatric psychiatrist has special skills in the management of acute schizophrenia-like disorders, the more severe mood disorders, severe anxiety and panic disorders, behavioral disorders resulting from dementing illness, complex personality and behavioral disturbances that interfere with appropriate medical management, and severe problems with sleep. Appropriate referral by the primary care physician to the geriatric psychiatrist, especially if initial therapy by the primary care physician proves ineffective, can both be cost-effective and provide relief of considerable suffering by the older adult with psychiatric impairment. **(p. 622)**

34.2 What is the major difficulty facing geriatric psychiatry fellowship training programs?

A. Prejudices about aging from younger physicians.
B. Lack of quality training programs.
C. Inadequate knowledge base for the field of geriatric psychiatry.
D. Low reimbursement for clinical services.
E. No certification examination like child psychiatry.

The correct response is option D.

Geriatric psychiatrists in the twenty-first century find themselves in a paradoxical situation. On the one hand, they are better trained, and their training rests on a firmer knowledge base, than at any time in the past. Of more importance, advances in understanding of the diagnosis and treatment of psychiatric disorders in late life have led to significantly improved and cost-effective therapies for older adults with psychiatric disorders. On the other hand, specialty care, in particular psychiatric care, could lose badly in the struggle for scarce health care resources. Administrators of fellowship programs in geriatric medicine as well as psychiatry are finding that recruitment to these programs has been more difficult in recent years. Training has never been better, and the original hesitation of many young physicians to treat older persons because of prejudices about aging has been largely overcome. Yet the uncertain future of medical specialties and the difficulty of receiving reimbursement for the care of older persons render geriatric medicine and geriatric psychiatry less desirable financially than procedure-driven medical specialties and primary care. **(p. 622)**

34.3 You admit one of your geriatric patients, who is covered by Medicare, to an inpatient psychiatric unit in the general hospital where you have admission privileges. The spouse asks you what Medicare will cover in terms of expenses. Which of the following is correct?

    A. Medicare has a 190-day lifetime psychiatric hospitalization limit for patients admitted to psychiatric units in general hospitals.
    B. There will be a one-time deductible of $768 for the first 60 days.
    C. Medicare does not pay after day 60 of a single hospitalization.
    D. There will be a daily co-pay for the first 60 days.
    E. Medicare does not reimburse patients for inpatient stays at freestanding psychiatric hospitals.

The correct response is option B.

Medicare requires a one-time deductible of $768 for a hospital stay of up to 60 days and daily deductibles after 60 days until the 150th day of a hospitalization, and Medicare does not pay after day 150 of a single hospitalization.

    Inpatient services have not been capitated in terms of reimbursement for individual hospitalizations, yet a 190-day lifetime psychiatric hospitalization limit remains in effect. This limit applies to freestanding psychiatric hospitals, not to psychiatric units in general hospitals. **(p. 623)**

34.4 Criteria that have been suggested as markers of successful aging include all of the following *except*

    A. Overall intelligence (IQ).
    B. Resiliency.
    C. Personal control.
    D. Life satisfaction.
    E. Adaptability.

The correct response is option A.

Criteria that have been suggested as markers of successful aging include length of life, biological health, life satisfaction and morale, cognitive efficacy, social competence and productivity, personal control, and resiliency and adaptivity (Baltes and Baltes 1990; Nowlin 1977, 1985; Palmore 1979; Rowe and Kahn 1987). Rowe and Kahn (1987) emphasized the need to explore how greatly extrinsic factors can play positive as well as negative roles in the aging process. For example, they noted studies of social support demonstrating that the availability of perceived connectedness and membership in a network of family and friends decreases the likelihood of illness and mortality (Berkman and Syme 1979; Blazer 1982). Rodin (1986) emphasized that older adults who had a greater sense of control over their environments had improved health and well-being compared with older adults who assumed a passive role toward their environments.

    Another theme that has traversed studies of successful aging is that of resiliency and adaptation. For example, Busse (1985) equated successful aging in part with the capacity to respond with resilience to challenges arising from changes within one's body, mind, and environment. A central task for older adults is to adopt effective strategies for dealing with losses and to be able to change goals and aspirations as either physical or psychosocial changes occur. **(pp. 624–625)**

34.5 Wisdom in successful aging has been defined by Baltes (1993). Which element of such wisdom does Baltes describe as "recognizing that no perfect solution exists"?

   A. Factual knowledge.
   B. Procedural knowledge.
   C. Lifespan contextualization.
   D. Value relativism.
   E. Acceptance of uncertainty.

The correct response is option E.

Baltes (1993) emphasized the importance of wisdom in successful aging. He suggested that wisdom includes 1) factual knowledge (the data necessary to respond to a situation); 2) procedural knowledge (strategies of acquiring data, making decisions, and providing advice); 3) lifespan contextualization (recognizing the inner relationships, tensions, and priorities of different life domains within the context of the life span); 4) value relativism (ability to separate one's own values from those of others); and 5) acceptance of uncertainty (recognizing that no perfect solution exists and optimizing the resolution of a situation as well as possible). Baltes noted that wisdom falls generally within the domain of cognitive pragmatics, or cognitive functioning that is primarily culture based and therefore potentially stable over time in persons who reach old age without specific brain pathology. In contrast, cognitive mechanics is roughly comparable to fluid intelligence and is primarily determined by the neurophysiological functioning of the brain. **(p. 625)**

References

Baltes PB: The aging mind: potential and limits. Gerontologist 33:580–594, 1993

Baltes PB, Baltes MM: Successful Aging: Perspectives From the Behavioral Sciences. New York, Cambridge University Press, 1990

Berkman LF, Syme LS: Social network, host resistance, and mortality: a 9-year follow-up study of Alameda County residents. Am J Epidemiol 109:186–204, 1979

Blazer DG: Social support and mortality in an elderly community population. Am J Epidemiol 115:684–694, 1982

Busse EW: Mental health and mental illness, in Normal Aging, III. Edited by Palmore E, Busse EW, Maddox G, et al. Durham, NC, Duke University Press, 1985, pp 81–91

Nowlin JB: Successful aging. Black Aging 2:4–6, 1977

Nowlin JB: Successful aging, in Normal Aging, III. Edited by Palmore E, Busse EW, Maddox G, et al. Durham, NC, Duke University Press, 1985, pp 34–46

Palmore E: Predictors of successful aging. Gerontologist 19:427–431, 1979

Rodin J: Aging and health: effects of the sense of control. Science 233:1271–1276, 1986

Rowe JW, Kahn RL: Human aging: usual and successful. Science 237:143–149